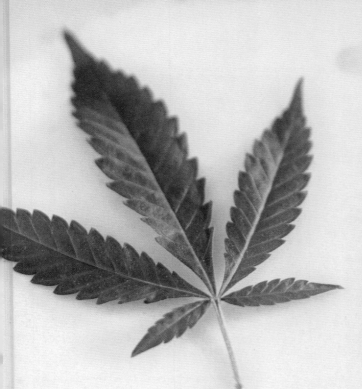

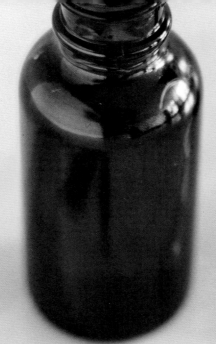

THE ULTIMATE GUIDE TO
CBD

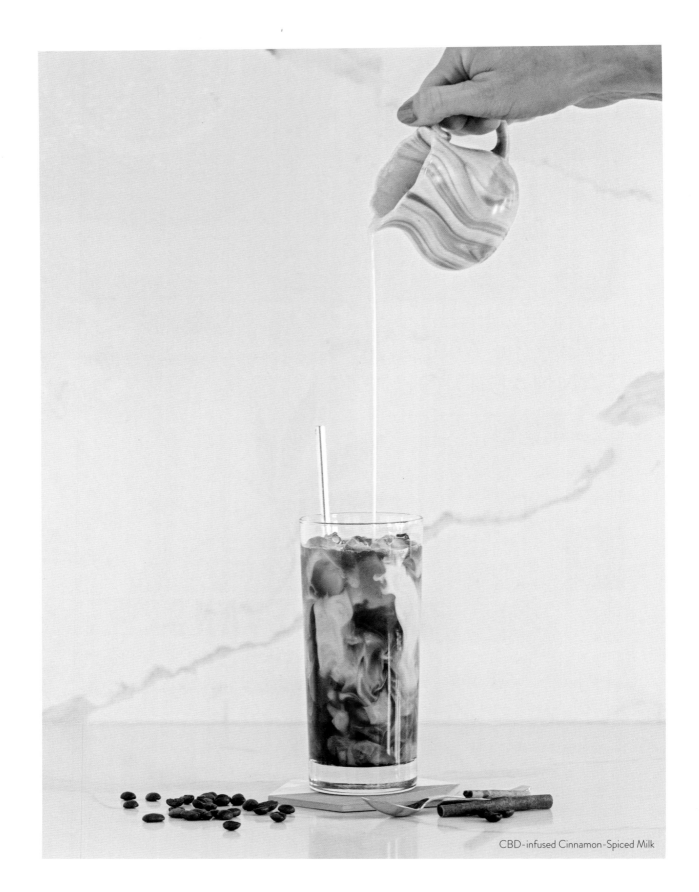

CBD-infused Cinnamon-Spiced Milk

CONTENTS

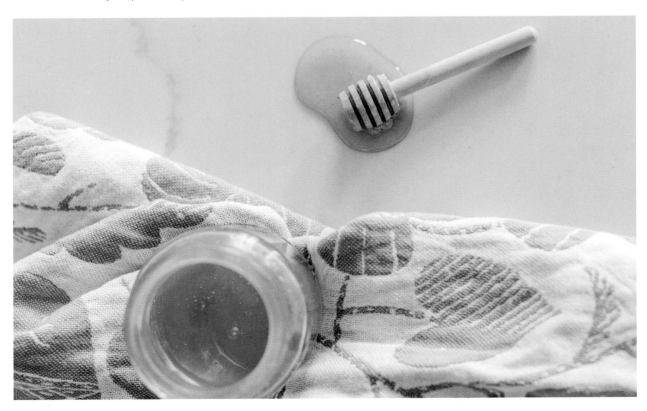

RECIPES

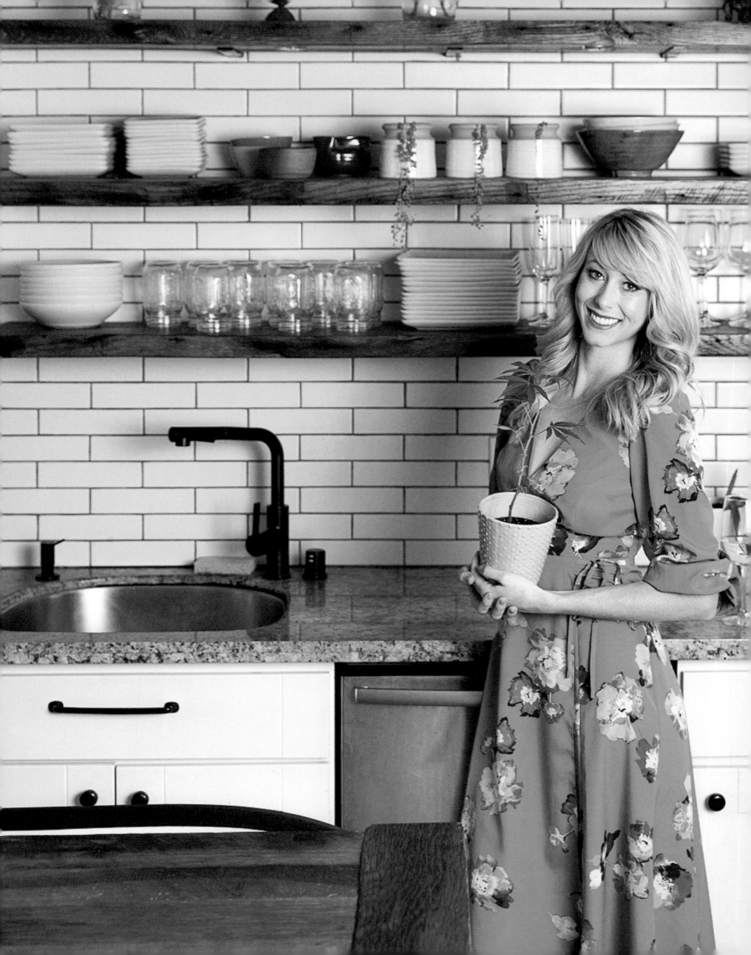

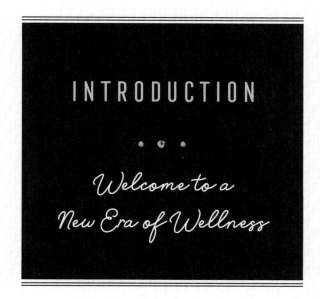

INTRODUCTION

• • •

Welcome to a
New Era of Wellness

Being active and finding new ways to stay healthy has always been a foundation for my way of thinking. When I was growing up in Truckee, California, my mother encouraged me to be my best self and to never forget to take care of my own personal well-being. Over the years, her insightful lessons in wellness inspired me to make health-conscious decisions, bringing a higher awareness to my lifestyle.

My mother was always the healthiest person I knew. She never missed her vitamins, knew far too much about supplements, never smoked, and could hike twenty miles without missing a beat. It was a devastating surprise when she was diagnosed with stage 4 non-small cell lung cancer in the fall of 2017. Everything I thought I knew about health was turned upside down.

A few months before receiving her diagnosis, I had launched my cannabis and lifestyle company, The Herb Somm. After experiencing a trauma of my own, I was using cannabis to help with sleep. Sensitive to products high in THC, I quickly became passionate about its counterpart, CBD, the powerful nonintoxicating cannabinoid that doesn't make you high.

For me, CBD was a game changer. It not only helped with my rest, but it brought me a sense of clarity and balance that improved my state of being. After learning about my mom's diagnosis, I wanted to focus my efforts on incorporating CBD into her life as well. After months of research, experimentation, and writing about this topic, CBD has played an important role in helping us both find stability.

I wrote *The Ultimate Guide to CBD* as a way to share everything I've learned along the way. This book will help you explore the different ways you can incorporate cannabidiol into your daily routines and rituals. For those of you interested in digging deeper, it also includes a variety of how-to guides and recipes. You can learn how to create your very own CBD tincture, bake CBD treats, mix a CBD latte, or craft a CBD massage oil.

For those of you just coming to CBD, yes, CBD stands for cannabidiol—a naturally occurring compound that's found in cannabis. Don't let that scare you away! Humans have had a long relationship with this sacred herb, dating back to more than 4,000 years ago in Asia where it was farmed for oil and for fiber. It was later used as herbal medicine more than 2,500 years ago. For centuries, our ancestors incorporated cannabis into their daily lives by combining it with different herbs to treat a variety of ailments. Cannabis was among those healing plants that provided a full spectrum of relief, but also played a role in deepening spirituality.

Since then, cannabis has found its way across many regions throughout the world. For those of you who live in the United States, cannabis and hemp cultivation played a significant role in the establishment of the nation. It was used to create fabric, rope, medicine, and more. The people of the United States loved the plant so much that it was printed on the ten-dollar bill as late as 1914.

Despite its cherished past, cannabis became criminalized, which led to prohibition in the United States. In the 1930s, the use of cannabis came under fire after the Federal Bureau of Narcotics was formed, headed by Harry J. Anslinger. Anslinger had it out for cannabis and he made it his mission to create propaganda that claimed cannabis was a dangerous substance that would make people commit crimes.

Because of these efforts during the "Reefer Madness" era, cannabis was later categorized as a "Schedule 1" drug when President Richard Nixon created the Drug Enforcement Administration (DEA). The DEA handles the enforcement of the drug schedule and oversees its changes. If you're not familiar with Schedule 1, the drugs that are listed in this category are the most dangerous substances around, containing no medicinal value with a high probability of abuse and addiction. This means that the federal government declared that cannabis was more dangerous than meth, cocaine, and oxycodone.

Unfortunately, these falsities plagued society for the past ninety years creating the stigma that surrounds cannabis. But there is a bright light at the end of the tunnel. Fast-forward to today. As more and more research and clinical studies are reaching the public eye, it is clear that cannabis has many medicinal benefits, as our ancestors knew long ago. Cannabis might also be a key to healthy living—with CBD at the forefront.

As you continue reading this book, you will discover that CBD is a powerful medicine, but it does not act alone. Cannabis contains a wealth of healing compounds that enhance each other when used together. If you've been following CBD, you might also be aware of something called hemp. Let me be clear: cannabis and hemp are the same plants. When you hear the term, "hemp" it is used to classify varieties of cannabis that contain less than

0.3 percent of THC by dry weight; however, there are different levels of quality within hemp. For the purposes of this book, when you come across this term, I am referring to organically grown therapeutic hemp, not industrial hemp. Flip to page 21 for a deeper dive into this topic.

You also might be wondering about the term, "marijuana." During the 1920s and 1930s the slang term "marihuana" and its variations was used by the U.S. government to classify high-resin cannabis strains that contained greater than 0.3 percent THC; however, it was also used to demonize and stigmatize immigrants and people of color who consumed cannabis recreationally during the Reefer Madness era. Knowing this, the plant's proper name—cannabis, not marijuana—will be used throughout this book.

As you can see, there is so much to learn about cannabis and what is soon to be your new wellness companion, cannabidiol. After doing countless hours of research and collaborating with some of the brightest thought leaders in the industry, this book contains a wealth of information that will enable you to use CBD successfully at home.

Before you begin this journey, I encourage you to set an intention and think about why you want to use cannabidiol in the first place. Are you feeling stressed? Are you looking for something to help with anxiety? Or are you simply curious to learn about the buzzword everyone is talking about? Whatever brought you here, write your intention down and focus on it as you work through each chapter. In the end, I hope that you'll discover that CBD can improve your mind, body, and spirit. Join me as we explore the wonderful world of cannabidiol.

With gratitude and love,

JAMIE EVANS, *The Herb Somm*

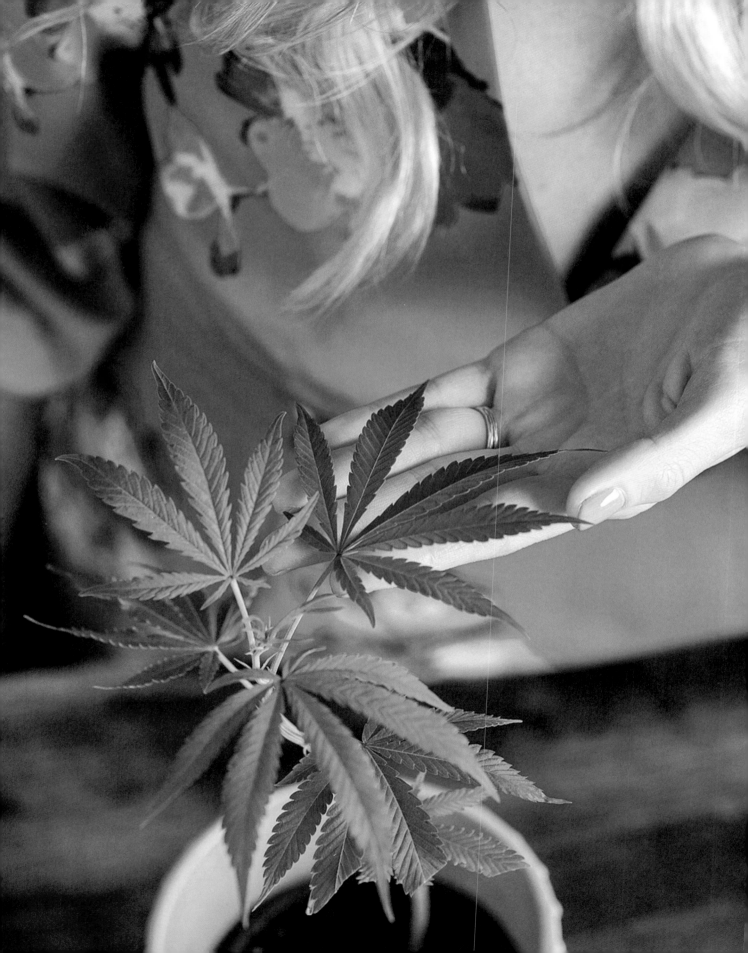

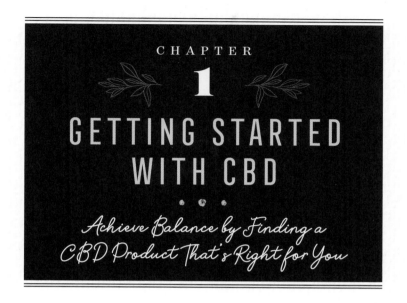

CHAPTER

1

GETTING STARTED WITH CBD

• • •

Achieve Balance by Finding a CBD Product That's Right for You

While the abundance of CBD products can seem overwhelming at first, once you know the basics of each category it's much easier to navigate the wide world of cannabidiol. By the end of this chapter, you will better understand how CBD works, learn about the various forms of CBD, and discover a selection of products that are right for you.

Keep in mind that CBD is not "one size fits all." It is an individualized treatment that is still in its youth when it comes to medical research. That said, you may need to experiment with different dosages, applications, and ratios to find your perfect balance. For some, this might include using a small dose of THC to improve CBD's effectiveness or using several different products for full-body therapy. For best results, you must also learn how to identify quality-made products. With a crowded market and lack of regulations, finding a safe and reliable CBD source is crucial.

The following pages will introduce you to some of the most common types of CBD as well as provide an overview of CBD's bioavailability rates, full-spectrum versus CBD isolates, how to choose a trustworthy CBD brand, and more. I encourage everyone to read this chapter, though if you find you already know the basics there's more for you in chapter 2!

THIS IS CBD

Simply defined, CBD (a.k.a. cannabidiol) is a natural compound that's found in cannabis. As a nonintoxicating and nonaddictive molecule, CBD is considered to be a phytocannabinoid—a cannabinoid or group of chemically similar compounds that are synthesized by plants—that works with hundreds of other important molecules to deliver enhanced therapeutic effects.

Miraculously, the ensemble of phytocannabinoids that has been identified in cannabis interact with cannabinoid receptors that are found in the human body.

The predominant active phytocannabinoids that you're probably most familiar with are THC and CBD. THC (delta-9-tetrahydrocannabinol) is the principal psychoactive component that gets you "high" when you consume cannabis. On the other hand, CBD (cannabidiol), does not produce the same sense of euphoria or mind-altering effects as THC, but it is indeed psychoactive. Because it can help reduce anxiety and relieve stress, CBD does interact with your brain in some capacity. It has been highly publicized that CBD is nonpsychoactive. Despite what many people claim, this is incorrect. Instead, it's best to think of it as "nonintoxicating."

While CBD and THC are the most widely known phytocannabinoids, there are more than one hundred different cannabinoid compounds that have been discovered in cannabis so far, although only a handful are present in high enough amounts to have any clinical impact on your health.

As you continue with this chapter, you will learn about the synergistic relationship that exists between CBD and THC, how CBD interacts with your body, CBD's healing benefits, how CBD impacts other medications, plus more. Learning these important details will help you as you begin your CBD journey.

CBD OR THC?

One of the biggest misconceptions that I've come across, particularly with beginners, is the belief that THC is bad and CBD is good (or a cure-all). The truth is both CBD and THC offer incredible healing benefits. When combined, these two powerful phytocannabinoids, alongside the other natural compounds discovered in cannabis, work together to enhance each other's efficacy so your body receives maximum therapeutic effects.

So how did THC get such an infamous reputation? If you look at the history of growing cannabis throughout the world, cannabis plants have similar amounts of THC and CBD, and have been used as an herbal medicine for centuries. However, the consumer desire for potent weed (meaning more THC-related effects) meant that the focus of breeding cannabis was pushed further and further toward maximizing THC. Strains were created to enhance the intoxicating effects, which, in turn, genetically decreased the medicinal value of cannabis, as CBD was reduced or altogether removed from the plant. Over the past few decades, these new strains dominated the market. Many people believed that cannabis was just about getting high—the movement toward THC-heavy strains reinforced this perception.

When we consider cannabis now—thanks to scientific discoveries and a greater focus on understanding how CBD and THC interact with our bodies—you should no longer feel like you have to choose one over the other. THC is *not* bad. The truth is, CBD and THC complement each other and work most efficiently when combined. These interactions are what make plant medicine so miraculous!

THE ENTOURAGE EFFECT

Cannabis is a botanical, and therefore it should be classified as a plant medicine. This means that the healing benefits that come from cannabis form from multiple compounds working together unlike pharmaceuticals that typically consist of one molecule. In other words, the whole plant is greater than the sum of its parts—it's a synergistic relationship that acts with an elevated effect. This phenomenon is known as the *entourage effect.*

Introduced by S. Ben-Shabat and Dr. Raphael Mechoulam in 1998, the entourage effect has become a pillar in cannabis research despite prohibitive federal restrictions that have generally prevented scientific studies on cannabis. During their early research, they discovered that phytocannabinoids such as CBD and THC, when combined with organic compounds known as terpenoids, work "in concert" or work as an "entourage" in a beneficial, harmonious way.

Unlike phytocannabinoids, terpenoids (also called terpenes) are not just found in cannabis. They can be found in many different herbs, spices, plants, flowers, etc., and offer a broad range of healing benefits. Plus, they are the driving source of cannabis' aromas and flavors, which make each strain unique in its own way. Research has shown that these compounds can enhance or alter the cannabinoid's medicinal properties. As popular cannabis education website *Leafly* explains, if THC and CBD are "the engine," terpenes are "the steering wheel and tires." You need all of these components in order for the car to run smoothly.

MEET THE OTHER COMMON CANNABINOIDS IN CANNABIS

In addition to CBD and THC, there are hundreds of other phytocannabinoids that are unique to cannabis, each offering different characteristics when interacting with our internal endocannabinoid systems. While THC and CBD are the most well studied and most prominent cannabinoids, below is an overview of some others that you might come across as you begin your cannabis journey.

CBC – Cannabichromene

Stemming from the same origins as both CBD and THC, CBC is a nonintoxicating cannabinoid that activates non-cannabinoid receptors in the body such as TRPV1 and TRPA1. Similar to CBD, CBC interacts with certain receptors that boost levels of endocannabinoids such as anandamide (AEA). CBC also acts as an anti-inflammatory, increases healthy brain function, and can potentially help treat acne.

CBDA – Cannabidiolic Acid

CBDA is the acidic precursor of CBD that's created by CBGA. CBDA does not interact with the usual elements of the endocannabinoid system, but it does produce anti-inflammatory effects similar to CBD. CBDA also acts as an anti-nausea supplement and could be an effective treatment for morning sickness. Leading cannabinoid researcher Dr. Michele Ross reports that it might also be better at lowering anxiety than CBD, at least in rodents. To integrate CBDA into your routine, try juicing raw CBD-rich cannabis leaves (unheated and not dried).

TABLE OF CANNABINOIDS

CBDV – Cannabidivarin

CBDV is a nonintoxicating cannabinoid that reduces the severity of seizures; therefore, it could be a suitable option for battling epilepsy. Research is also indicating that CBDV can potentially reduce or eliminate nausea associated with several conditions.

CBG – Cannabigerol

CBG is a lesser-known nonintoxicating cannabinoid that's not widely present in most strains. Beginning as CBGA or cannabigerolic acid, cannabis plants produce this cannabinoid that later turns into THCA, CBDA, or CBCA, depending on the enzymes that make up the plant. While difficult to capture on its own, CBG acts as an anti-inflammatory, anti-anxiety, antibacterial, as well as produces other positive calming side effects.

CBN – Cannabinol

If you're looking for a good night's rest, CBN might be your new best friend. Produced by the oxidation of THC and degradation from heat and light after the flower is harvested, CBN is mildly intoxicating and is best known for its sedative side effects. If you've ever consumed an old bag of weed and felt really tired, pronounced levels of CBN could be the culprit. Besides the sedative effects, CBN can be used as a mild pain reliever and act as an appetite stimulant.

THC – Tetrahydrocannabinol

I know that you've already learned a little bit about THC, but given its importance, there is more ground to cover. Delta-9-tetrahydrocannabinol is the primary intoxicating component of cannabis that's created when THCA is exposed to heat via decarboxylation. Found in several different variations, THC binds directly to CB1 and CB2 receptors delivering a broad range of therapeutic benefits including pain relief, anti-inflammation, anti-nausea, acts as a sleep aid, plus more. If overconsumed, THC can present some unpleasant side effects such as paranoia. For beginners, combine THC with CBD for best results.

THCA – Tetrahydrocannabinolic Acid

THCA is the nonintoxicating acid form of THC that's created by CBGA. It is the most prominent compound that's found in raw cannabis. Unlike THC, THCA doesn't appear to cross the blood-brain barrier and only activates receptors in the body, not the brain. Because it's nonintoxicating, THCA is quickly gaining popularity and provides many health benefits. For example, THCA can increase the appetite and reduce nausea and vomiting. It also acts as a powerful anti-inflammatory and pain reliever without the euphoria of THC. Because THCA converts to THC via decarboxylation, it's best to keep TCHA products away from heat and store in a cool place if you wish to consume the cannabinoid in its in nonintoxicating form.

THCV – Tetrahydrocannabivarin

Quickly gaining the attention of those seeking an option for weight loss, THCV is a variation of THC that is known to suppress the appetite. Because of its interaction with CB1 receptors, THCV reduces feelings that evoke hunger and presents some intoxicating effects. THCV can also be somewhat stimulating, so it might not be effective for sleep.

CBD & YOUR BODY

While research on cannabis is still in the early stages, there are a few important discoveries on how and why CBD, THC, and the other phytocannabinoids can improve your health. It all comes down to the endocannabinoid system and the natural cannabinoids that are already in your body. Here's how it all works:

✳ Cannabis is a plant that naturally interacts with your biological system as the molecules within the plant work with different sites that are found throughout the body. With the discovery of the endocannabinoid system (ECS), we realized phytocannabinoids, such as CBD and THC, are able to stimulate different receptors that help maintain homeostasis (your happy place) by regulating appetite, mood, memory, inflammation, and more.

✳ In addition to phytocannabinoids, humans and mammals produce their own cannabinoids in the body and the brain. These endogenous cannabinoids, called *endocannabinoids,* interact with your endocannabinoid system in the same way that phytocannabinoids do. In fact, the endocannabinoid system was made for endocannabinoids, but we can supplement with phytocannabinoids to keep the ECS balanced.

✳ Both humans and mammals experience endocannabinoid deficiencies, which can greatly impact your health, causing a long list of ailments. Dr. Michele Ross explains that endocannabinoid deficiency can feel a lot like burnout, and that's because the endocannabinoid system is often depleted when we are experiencing chronic stress. To rebalance your endocannabinoid system, phytocannabinoids can be integrated into your daily health routine to restore the endocannabinoids that have been diminished. In other words, cannabis and hemp products can be important supplements that can enhance your body's internal system. There's a reason cannabis has been used as a medicine for centuries.

THE ENDOCANNABINOID SYSTEM

Let's take a closer look at the endocannabinoid system. All vertebrate species, which include both humans and all other mammals, have endocannabinoid systems that help maintain homeostasis. The ECS is a biological system that's composed of different endocannabinoids, cannabinoid receptors, and enzymes that are expressed throughout the body. It is the largest neurotransmitter system with cannabinoid receptors found on cells in the central nervous system (consisting of the brain and spinal cord), reproductive system, immune system, tissue, glands, and more.

The ECS keeps your mind and body in check and in balance. It plays a critical role in regulating several physiological processes including your appetite, mood, pain, blood pressure, memory, hormones, and more. It also helps your body deal with stress, which can greatly impact your health over time.

The endocannabinoid system consists of three main components: *cannabinoid receptors* such as the CB1 and CB2 receptors that are found on the surface of cells, *endocannabinoids* or cannabinoid signaling molecules that activate cannabinoid receptors, and *metabolic cannabinoid enzymes* that synthesize and break down endocannabinoids after they are used. Let's explore this on a deeper level.

CANNABINOID RECEPTORS: CB1 & CB2 RECEPTORS

Two important elements of the endocannabinoid system include cannabinoid receptors CB1 and CB2, which are classified as G protein-coupled receptors (GPCRs) that modulate neurotransmitters such as endocannabinoids and phytocannabinoids. CB1 receptors are found in the brain and body and are activated by endocannabinoids anandamide (AEA) and 2-arachidonoyl glycerol (2-AG) as well as phytocannabinoids such as THC. These important receptors are also impacted by the release of other important neurotransmitters in the brain including serotonin, dopamine, histamine, endorphins, and more. CB1 also helps regulate anxiety, pain relief, mood, and happiness; when balanced, our body is in homeostasis. When you use a product that contains THC, CB1 receptors are what THC binds to or activates to produce the "high" feeling that's associated with consuming cannabis. You can think of CB1 as a lock and THC as a key as they fit together.

CB2 receptors are primarily found on the cells of the immune system—but also in the organs, bones, and brain. CB2 receptors are activated by AEA, 2-AG, and THC, but also by the terpene beta-Caryophyllene, plus other molecules. When CB2 is activated by compounds such as THC, it does not produce intoxicating effects, which are frequently observed with CB1 receptors. Instead, CB2 receptors help modulate inflammation and pain, help our immune response to pathogens, and protect against bone loss in the body as we age.

While THC binds directly to both cannabinoid receptors, CBD is a different story. Cannabidiol does not interact with CB1 or CB2 receptors directly, but interacts in an indirect way. For example, CBD blocks THC from binding to CB1 receptors, therefore, blunting THC's intoxicating effects. Thus, someone would not feel as "stoned" when they use a product that contains both CBD and THC versus a product that only contains THC. CBD also has the ability to alter and/or improve the capabilities of non-cannabinoid receptors (such as serotonin 5-HT1A and vanilloid receptor TRPV1), interacting with GABA-A receptors to calm the central nervous system, and deactivate G protein-coupled receptor GPR55, which is associated with osteoporosis and bone reabsorption. Last but not least, CBD increases the levels of endocannabinoid AEA, which means more feelings of joy, happiness, and pleasure. Who wouldn't want that?

ENDOCANNABINOIDS: ANANDAMIDE (AEA) & 2-ARACHIDONOYL GLYCEROL (2-AG)

Like phytocannabinoids, our natural endocannabinoids interact with the endocannabinoid system. Two of the primary endocannabinoids are AEA and 2-AG. These endocannabinoids are not stored in the body, but are produced "on demand" by fatty acid proteins. Once they are created, they interact with the body locally where they were synthesized and activate CB1 and CB2 receptors.

AEA is a cannabinoid-signaling molecule that's created in the brain. It is often known as the "bliss molecule." This type of fatty acid neurotransmitter binds to cannabinoid receptors throughout the body to produce a state of heightened happiness. It's also an important element in memory, motivation, higher thought processes, and movement control. 2-AG is also found in the brain and was discovered after scientists identified AEA. While 2-AG binds to both CB1 and CB2 receptors, it also interacts with the TRPV1 (transient receptor potential vanilloid type one) and other receptors that regulate pain, body temperature, anxiety, memory, and more.

Together, AEA and 2-AG work as a power team to activate the most important receptor sites to protect the brain and body, while keeping your internal system in equilibrium.

METABOLIC CANNABINOID ENZYMES

Another important piece to the ECS puzzle are metabolic cannabinoid enzymes that either synthesize or break down endocannabinoids AEA and 2-AG. AEA is mostly impacted by the NAPE enzyme, which produces AEA in the brain, and the FAAH enzyme, which breaks down AEA after it's done being used. On the other hand, 2-AG is mostly impacted by the DAGL enzyme, which synthesizes 2-AG in the brain, and the MAGL enzyme, which breaks it down. Both the FAAH and MAGL enzymes are important because they ensure that endocannabinoids get used when they are needed, but not for more than what's necessary. This process helps keep our body in check.

As you can see, the endocannabinoid system is a complex system, and researchers are just in the early stages of fully understanding how all of the components work. However, one thing we do know for sure is that by supplementing phytocannabinoids such as CBD and THC into your daily health care routine, you can bring balance back to your ECS by restoring the cannabinoids that have been depleted.

HEMP-DERIVED CBD VS. CANNABIS-DERIVED CBD

featuring Charlotte Palermino, cannabis educator & co-founder of Nice Paper

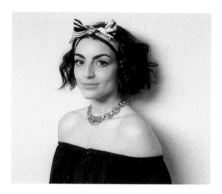

Charlotte Palermino is the co-founder of Nice Paper, a high-design publishing platform. In addition to brand consulting for cannabis companies in Canada and the United States, Nice Paper publishes a weekly newsletter that explores the people and products of weed alongside experts in the space that are on the frontier of what's to come. In addition to Nice Paper, Charlotte is the CEO of Dieu X, a cannabinoid skin care line. Follow Charlotte @charlotteparler and @itsnicepaper or visit benicepaper.com

Charlotte Palermino: "At the end of the day, a cannabinoid is a cannabinoid. In the case of CBD or cannabidiol, it doesn't matter if it comes from a hemp plant or a cannabis plant as long as they are farmed and processed the same way. When it comes to CBD there is no difference between cannabis and therapeutic hemp. The only place they differ is in terpene composition and another important cannabinoid concentration, THC or tetrahydrocannabinol; however, industrial hemp is a different story. Because production is primarily focused on fiber and seed oil, industrial hemp has been known to contain fewer cannabinoids and terpenes by dry weight, but the CBD it does contain is the same CBD molecule that's found in cannabis.

Repeat: cannabis CBD isn't better or worse than hemp CBD; it's the same chemical compound. THC is the only place where these plants diverge in federal regulation, as hemp has to legally have less than 0.3 percent THC. Anything more? It's weed.

When you isolate CBD, you can't tell if it comes from hemp or cannabis. When it comes to full-spectrum CBD (i.e., a CBD product that contains a "full spectrum" of cannabinoids, terpenes, etc., versus a product where just the CBD is stripped out; think vitamin C pill versus a glass of orange juice), I always recommend, when possible, to buy from an extremely reputable source—or buy from a licensed dispensary as cannabis is much more regulated than hemp. When navigating the unregulated CBD market always ask for a Certificate of Analysis (COA) for the batch you are buying. Also keep an eye out for other cannabinoids such as CBN, which can be sedative, CBC, which can help with inflammation, and CBG. CBD is just one cannabinoid. The exciting thing with cannabis is how much more we have to learn in the coming years!"

FULL SPECTRUM, BROAD SPECTRUM & CBD ISOLATES

If you've been doing your research, you might have come across the terms full spectrum, broad spectrum, and CBD isolate. What do these phrases mean and why do they matter so much?

As you learned earlier, there is a powerful relationship between CBD and the other natural compounds that are found in cannabis. By working together, the "entourage" of these therapeutic components is what provides our bodies with optimal healing benefits.

The most effective CBD products are whole-plant derived products that contain a "full spectrum" of CBD, THC, CBN, CBG, CBC, plus other phytocannabinoids, terpenes, flavonoids, and fatty acids. While these products do contain THC, some might only have trace amounts; therefore, they do not impart intoxicating effects. The key thing here is knowing that the product does contain THC, which is actually the most beneficial way to consume CBD. Remember, the synergy and interactions that exist between all of the plant's compounds are known to provide the best results because they enhance each other.

Broad-spectrum and isolates are other common terms that are used to describe CBD products. If you're someone concerned about THC showing up in a drug test or you simply don't want to consume it, broad-spectrum hemp products are your best option. Unlike full-spectrum, they don't contain THC, so they're not classified as "whole-plant" items. Broad-spectrum CBD products go through extra processing to remove all traces of THC while focusing on preserving the other cannabinoids and terpenes.

CBD isolates are another story. As the name suggests, CBD isolate products are made from "isolated" CBD, where the CBD compound is extracted and separated from the rest of the plant. This means that all of the other healing cannabinoids, terpenes, waxes, and oils are removed, leaving you with 99+% pure CBD. While pure CBD might sound like a good thing, it's not the best form of medicine because you are losing all of the beneficial attributes of the entourage effect. However, isolates can offer some value for those who are sensitive to THC or for those living in places where full-spectrum products are not available.

Knowing this, it's up to you to decide what method works best to suit your personal needs and concerns. This book provides different ways that you can create CBD self-care products, cuisine, and beverages using all three options.

THE BIOAVAILABILITY OF CBD

As you begin to explore CBD products, understanding bioavailability rates is crucial if you want to maximize the effectiveness of your CBD. Bioavailability refers to the degree and rate at which a substance is absorbed into the bloodstream. For example, when a medication is introduced into your body via intravenous therapy (a.k.a. an IV), its bioavailability is considered 100 percent because all of the medication has been integrated directly into the bloodstream.

When a medication is taken through other routes (inhalation, oral consumption, ingestion, etc.), bioavailability rates decrease because the medicine or active compound, in this case CBD, either doesn't get fully absorbed or it must be metabolized and digested before effects sets in. This phenomenon is known as the "first pass effect." The first pass effect occurs when a medication is greatly reduced in concentration after its metabolized, therefore, decreasing its effectiveness after it passes through the gut and liver before it reaches the bloodstream. While the first pass effect has an influence on CBD, this is not the same case for THC. When ingested orally, THC converts to 11-hydroxy-THC, which can actually produce stronger effects. Turn to page 24 for a deeper look into smoking versus eating/drinking THC and CBD products.

When it comes to cannabis, bioavailability rates are influenced by the method of usage and the product itself. Theoretically, full-spectrum products help improve bioavailability due to the interactions that improve CBD's efficacy (the entourage effect); however, depending on how you consume CBD, its effectiveness can vary. In general, studies are showing that smoking, vaping, sublingual applications, and rectal suppositories deliver the highest bioavailability rates. Edibles, pills, and capsules are among the lowest. In the coming pages, you will learn about each consumption category and bioavailability rate in greater detail.

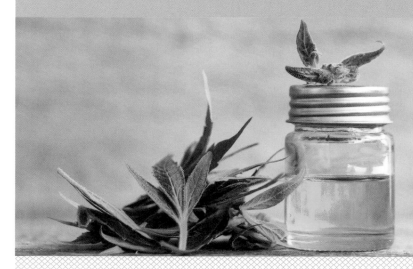

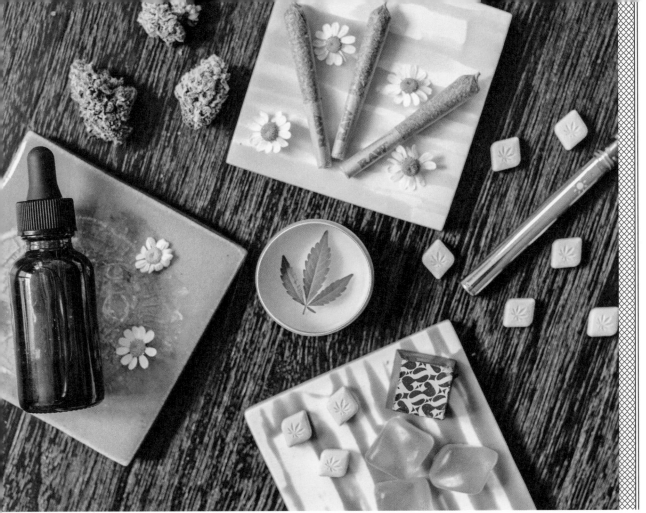

Clockwise, from top:
CBD-rich prerolls, Kiva
Confections Petra Mints,
TSO Sonoma Mindful
Pen, Garden Society
Milk Chocolates, Kiva
Confections Camino
Sparkling Pear Gummies,
Herb Somm tincture, and
CBD-rich flower

HOW TO USE CBD

There are many, many ways that you can enjoy CBD without having to be an expert. Because cannabidiol is a nonintoxicating compound, it is much easier to navigate than products infused with THC because you are not at risk of getting overly high when experimenting with differ-ent forms. Depending on what your needs are, the most common delivery methods include inhaling CBD via smoking or vaping (see more about vaping on page 28), ingesting CBD or taking it sublingually, applying CBD topically or through a transdermal patch, and taking CBD via a suppository.

Keep in mind that onset times, duration of effects, and bioavailability rates differ between each method and type of product. There is also currently no standard for dosing CBD (see more on page 31), so figuring out what works best for your own body should be a priority when first experimenting with cannabis or hemp products.

Reactions to CBD vary from person to person—it is a very personalized medicine. If some-thing works well for your best friend or significant other, be aware that it might not work well for you. This means that you might have to try a few different types of applications to achieve the best results, so be sure to keep an open mind and don't be afraid to try something new.

It's also very important to be aware that CBD is not like THC. You might not perceive any noticeable effects when it's absorbed into your body. For this reason, I recommend thinking of CBD more like a vitamin. Although you might not feel much psychologically, there is something happening inside your body physiologically. That said, CBD helps take the edge off for some. If you are feeling stressed out or anxious, CBD might help you feel more relaxed and centered. If your body is feeling sore and achy, CBD might provide a sense of relief because of its powerful anti-inflammatory effects.

Before using CBD, it's best to determine why you want to take it and then figure out how you're going to integrate it into your routine based on your particular needs. To help with the discovery process, here is a list of some of the most common delivery methods.

INGESTION & ORAL CONSUMPTION

If you're not big on smoking or vaping, consuming CBD as a beverage, capsule, edible, lozenge, sublingual, or tincture is a popular way to integrate cannabidiol into your routine. In general, the bioavailability of CBD products in these categories tends to fall between 6 and 20 percent; however, sublinguals can reach between 12 and 35 percent. If you're planning on eating an edible or something else that requires digestion, be aware that it can take up to 2 hours or more for effects to kick in, although this will be very subtle for CBD.

While infused foods and beverages are fun for recreational purposes, they are probably not the best options for serious medical conditions. Instead, there are other forms of oral consumption products that do not have to be digested that have higher bioavailability rates, including tinctures, tablinguals, and sublingual strips. Compared to inhalation, the most prominent differences are the bioavailability rates and the delayed onset of effects when CBD or THC is ingested or consumed orally.

CBD Beverages

CBD beverages are quickly becoming a popular way to consume cannabis and hemp products. In addition to trendy cocktails and mocktails, you can also find canned or bottled CBD drinks that are most often made into sparkling beverages. Most CBD and THC beverage companies are using nanotechnology to integrate cannabinoids into drinks by making compounds, such as CBD, water-suspended. This allows the CBD or THC to be integrated into a beverage seamlessly without leaving behind residue or separating like a salad dressing. After consuming an infused beverage, effects set in more quickly than with food, so you might start noticing effects around 20 to 45 minutes, depending on your body. Turn to chapter 4 for an in-depth exploration of CBD and beverages.

Capsules & Supplements

Taking CBD in a capsule or supplement is another way to consume plant medicine, and it is an effective way to determine a precise dose. Containing pure CBD oil or a powdered blend, CBD capsules and supplements typically take around 30 to 60 minutes to kick in, but can last for a long time depending on the dose consumed. Bioavailability rates run on the lower side, similar to other forms of digestible products; however, these products are quickly becoming a favorite for athletes as they provide some unique benefits. Flip to page 67 for more information on how you can integrate CBD capsules into your fitness routine.

Edibles

Consuming cannabidiol via premade edible products is a growing trend. They taste great and can be a pleasurable way to begin your CBD journey. The trick to any edible experience is to "start slow, go low." Be patient after you eat an edible and begin with a low dose—especially when it comes to THC. While CBD won't give you a head change or pronounced effects, you will definitely know when a THC edible sets in, which can take anywhere from 45 minutes up to 2 hours or more.

You must be patient and be aware of your own metabolism when eating edibles or infused cuisine. For beginners, I usually recommend starting with 15 to 30 milligrams of CBD or 1 to 5 milligrams of THC for your first edible experience and see how it goes. Turn to page 146 to read more about how to eat edibles and infused foods safely and responsibly.

Lozenges

CBD lozenges are small medicinal tablets, similar to cough drops or hard candy, that are dissolved in the mouth. Because the medicine is absorbed through membranes in your mouth and delivered to the bloodstream, effects can set in as fast as 20 minutes.

Sublingual Products

Sublingual products refer to any product that you place under your tongue to be absorbed through the oral mucosal membranes in your mouth including strips, sprays, oils, tablinguals, and tinctures. To do so successfully, place the CBD sublingual product or a few drops of CBD oil under your tongue and hold it there for a minute or two before swallowing. Compared to other forms of oral consumption, sublinguals have some of the highest bioavailability rates because they are absorbed into the bloodstream so quickly. They're also one of the best ways to increase the bioavailability of all of the other important cannabinoids such as THC.

Tinctures and CBD oils are a great smoke-free option that are convenient, discreet, and can be taken sublingually or mixed into food or drinks. They are also ideal for customizing dosages, which are easily administered by the use of a measured dropper. Turn to page 31 to learn more.

TOPICALS & TRANSDERMAL PATCHES

Topicals, such as CBD lotion, balms, and salves, are great options for targeting specific trouble areas on the body and work by absorbing through the skin. Transdermal patches offer a solution for deep, long-lasting full-body relief as CBD or THC penetrate all skin layers, reaching the bloodstream and circulating throughout the body.

Note: While it may seem extreme, suppositories offer some of the highest bioavailability rates (in some cases up to 80 percent). This method is popular among medical patients as medicine fully absorbs into the body via rectal or vaginal tissue. Suppositories also allow patients to take higher doses of THC without experiencing enhanced intoxicating effects or a "head high" because they offer a direct application to the bloodstream bypassing the liver— the liver is one of the major components that contributes to euphoric or "high" feelings.

INHALATION

Whether you are smoking or vaping, inhaling CBD is one of the most common and efficient ways to consume cannabidiol with effects lasting up to 2 hours or more. By introducing CBD into your body through the lungs, cannabidiol reaches the bloodstream delivering high bioavailability rates (around 30 percent), making it one of the most effective ways to get CBD into your body. However, be aware that smoking can cause other health issues, so this method is not recommended for everyone.

Smoking CBD-rich Flower

When in doubt, smoking dry cannabis flower is the tried-and-true method of consuming cannabis that has been practiced for ages. There are many methods that you can use to smoke CBD-rich flower including rolling a joint or blunt, lighting up a preroll, using a glass piece (such as a pipe, bubbler, or bong), or by using a dry flower vaporizer. Depending on what method you choose, the most important part of consuming dry flower is to make sure it is clean, pesticide-free cannabis. The best place to find high-quality flower is at a licensed dispensary. You can rest assured that the flower has gone through rigorous testing to ensure that what you're buying is pure, clean cannabis. If you're thinking about smoking hemp flower, make sure that you're sourcing clean, organic therapeutic hemp and not industrial hemp. Depending on how it's grown, industrial hemp can be packed with contaminants that you do not want to inhale.

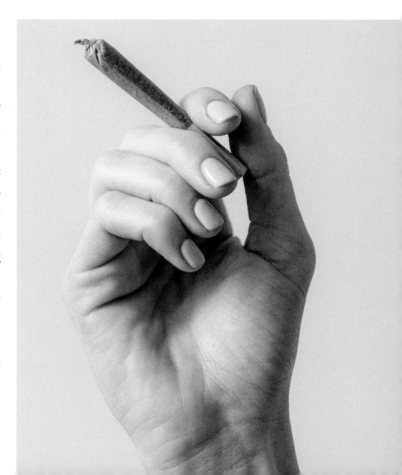

Vaping

Vaporizers are a popular choice for inhaling cannabis because they are discrete and convenient. Compared to traditional methods of smoking, vaporizers are thought to be a healthier option because you're not combusting the flower, which eliminates the dangerous by-products of smoke; however, it's imperative that you know where your products are coming from and that they are tested for dangerous additives, chemicals, and pesticides. Only purchase from licensed dispensaries that carry trusted brands.

Vaporizers work by heating cannabis flower, oil, or concentrates by conduction (heating by direct contact with a heat source) or convection (heating a material with hot air blown through a heating element.) There are pros and cons to both methods, but in general, the convection method is preferred for vaping flowers because it best preserves terpene profiles.

If you consider yourself to be an expert, or a "cannabis connoisseur," then convection is a good option for you. If you're looking for something more user friendly, conduction vaporizers might be a good option. There are also a number of vape pens that are designed for beginners. Some of the most popular trending vapes are named after the intended effect you'll perceive after using them, such as Bliss, Sleep, Calm, or Relief.

A Note on Vaping

If you're curious to explore vaporizers further, be aware that there are some precautions you should take before experimenting. At the time of this writing, many of the vaping illnesses that have swept across the United States have been traced back to products that were created and purchased through the illicit market—not through legal, licensed dispensaries. Here are some tips to help you shop smarter:

✳ Never trust something that is suspiciously underpriced.

✳ If the product doesn't contain a Certificate of Analysis (COA), move on.

✳ Do your research online to ensure the company or dispensary you're purchasing from is legitimate and licensed.

✳ Pay close attention to the ingredients listed on the packaging. Do not ingest anything that is not pure plant extract and watch out for dangerous additives such as vitamin E acetate, MCT oil, and propylene glycol. You do not want these substances in your lungs!

While all of these things might sound intimidating, remember that there are also many trusted and responsible brands that care about their products and customers. Flip to the Resources on page 206 to see a listing of my favorite vaporizer products. If vaping is not for you, don't worry. As you've learned, there are many other ways you can enjoy cannabis and CBD.

CBD'S THERAPEUTIC EFFECTS

In addition to CBD's ability to boost the blissful endocannabinoid anandamide (AEA), it also has the ability to influence a wide range of other molecules and receptor systems in the brain and body to produce a wide range of therapeutic effects. For instance, CBD acts as a powerful anti-inflammatory by inhibiting the release of inflammatory cytokines or signaling molecules excreted from immune cells that promote inflammation in the body. If you experience anxiety, CBD interacts with serotonin receptors in the brain to produce anti-anxiety effects. Did I mention it can improve skin conditions such as acne? Yup, it's true. CBD is also a powerful antioxidant. In fact, there's research that suggests that CBD is even more effective than vitamins C and E as a neuroprotective antioxidant.

CBD might aid those who suffer from PTSD and insomnia, and it interacts with the opioid receptors in the brain that help regulate pain. These receptors are the primary targets of pharmaceutical pain killers, making CBD (and THC) medications a potential solution for replacing dangerous opioid pills as well as helping stop addiction. Cannabis should not be considered as the entry drug, but rather an exit tool that provides new options for care.

In addition, there is scientific evidence that CBD is effective for treating childhood epilepsy syndromes, such as Dravet syndrome and Lennox-Gastaut syndrome, which usually don't respond to traditional antiseizure medications. When treated with CBD, the results were so drastic that the FDA approved the first cannabis-derived medicine, Epidiolex, which contains high amounts of CBD for oral consumption.

NOTE

While CBD does provide many benefits, it's important to remember that it's not a cure-all. For those considering taking it for more serious health issues, such as cancer, be sure to consult with a trained health care professional. CBD has the ability to either enhance or inhibit the way other medications work in your body, which can cause other health issues. That said, it's extremely important to notify your doctor, especially if you are not aware of how CBD will interact with the other pharmaceutical drugs that you might be taking.

As a rule of thumb, if your medication bottle has a warning label that says, "Do Not Consume with Grapefruit," you should probably not be taking CBD with that medication either because CBD and grapefruit are known to interact with certain drugs that impact important enzymes in your liver. See more on CBD and medications on page 30. Even though CBD is nonintoxicating and it has few known adverse side effects, it's best to proceed with caution, especially with the lack of regulations in testing CBD products.

CBD & OTHER MEDICATIONS

featuring Dr. Michele Ross, Ph.D., CEO of Infused Health

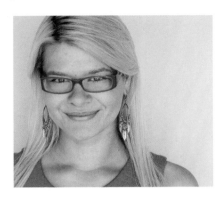

Dr. Michele Ross, Ph.D., M.B.A., is a neuroscientist and health coach with a passion to help patients with chronic illnesses live their best life. Dr. Ross is both a cannabinoid medicine researcher and a cannabis patient. After being diagnosed with fibromyalgia, neuropathy, and chronic pelvic pain, cannabis and kratom were the only treatments that reduced her symptoms and allowed her to return to work. In 2013, she founded the Endocannabinoid Deficiency Foundation, later known as IMPACT Network, which was the first nonprofit to provide research and advocacy on cannabis for women's health. In 2017, she founded Infused Health, an online platform for cannabis education and health coaching. Dr. Ross is also the celebrated author of Vitamin Weed: A 4-Step Plan to Prevent and Reverse Endocannabinoid Deficiency. *Follow Dr. Michele Ross @drmicheleross or visit www.drmicheleross.com.*

Dr. Michele Ross: "If you're thinking about taking CBD while on other medications take precautions. Unfortunately, CBD is a potent inhibitor of two types of p450 liver and gut enzymes that break down over a third of prescription drugs. These two types of p450 enzymes are CYP3A4 and CYP2DC. If you're using CBD with a drug that is metabolized by CYP3A4 or CYP2DC, the drug stays in your system longer. This can be dangerous because this could amplify the side effects of the drug like sleepiness, nausea, headache, blood thinning, or other serious issues. Many common drugs such as antidepressants, antiseizure drugs, and blood thinners have reported interactions with CBD. And just because a drug has not had a published drug interaction, it doesn't mean that it hasn't happened, it just means the research into it hasn't been funded.

I always recommend that patients talk with their doctor or other health professionals if they are on prescription medication before using CBD, especially at doses higher than 10 milligrams of CBD a day. At Infused Health, one of the things we do is review a patient's medical history for potential drug interactions, and then suggest that the dosage of medication be lowered with their doctor's approval, or switch to a different cannabinoid, such as THC, that doesn't have the same drug interaction.

If you're thinking about using CBD, talk to a professional about using cannabis for medical purposes. It's not as easy as smoking a joint and your pain goes away. Each patient has a unique medical history, genetics, liver, etc., that will require a different approach to cannabis treatment. Invest in a cannabis coach or cannabis nurse to help you save money that would be wasted on buying the wrong products and to help you get back to health faster."

Dabbing

If you're brand new to cannabis, you probably shouldn't start with dabbing, but it's not as scary as you may think. If you're looking for a very potent way to medicate, dabbing incorporates highly condensed forms of cannabis, such as wax, shatter, or budder, and a special apparatus called a "dab rig" to heat up powerful concentrates for inhalation.

You should always take precautions before dabbing and know your limits. If you're dabbing THC, be aware that you might get really, really stoned, which can produce overwhelming feelings if you're not prepared for it; however, some people find great relief dabbing THC, so it really depends on how your body handles concentrated levels of the compound. You can also dab CBD concentrates, which do not have the same intoxicating effects as THC. If done correctly and safely, dabbing is a reliable way to get a very high dose of CBD into your body quickly.

INTRODUCTION TO DOSING

Now that you know the many ways to use CBD, let's talk about dosing. Because cannabis is an individualized form of medicine (i.e., not "one size fits all"), there are no standards for how many milligrams a person should consume. An "accurate dose" completely depends on the person taking the plant medicine and is influenced by many factors including metabolism, body weight, diet, etc.

In the cannabis world, a dose refers to how much CBD, THC, CBN, or other active compounds are in your products. While research is showing that CBD is safe when consumed at higher doses, it is best to start on the lower side of the dosage range and adjust upward over time until the desired effect is achieved. Start low, go slow. If you have access to cannabis products that contain both CBD and THC, modify the amount of CBD and THC you are taking until you find a ratio that works best for you. Remember, a higher ratio of CBD to THC means you'll have less of a high.

Below are some other recommendations on how to find your ideal dose:

✻ When experimenting with different types of CBD, if you are using a professionally made product, start with the manufacturer's recommended dose per serving. CBD products and potency can vary from brand to brand, so begin with what the manufacturer suggests first. Before mixing it into a recipe, try a single serving of the CBD on its own. After consuming, see how you feel and then go up or down in milligrams depending on your needs.

✻ If you're ready to increase the dosage, begin increasing your dose by 25 percent increments over time. Some of the best CBD oils come with labeled increments of 0.25 milliliters on the dropper (0.25 ml, 0.50 ml, 0.75 ml), so it's easy to track your progress. Be sure to take notes of how you're feeling as your milligram intake increases.

✳ Know the difference between hemp-derived CBD and cannabis-derived CBD. When using hemp-derived CBD, you don't need to worry about the CBD:THC ratio as much, but if you're using a cannabis-derived CBD oil with higher levels of THC, make sure to factor in both phytocannabinoids into your milligram count as you begin to increase or decrease your dosage. If you increase the CBD, you're increasing the THC.

✳ If you live in a state where you have access to cannabis-derived CBD, don't be afraid to go to your local licensed dispensary and pick up products. Budtenders are knowledgeable, friendly, and there to help you choose the best items based on your needs. You'll find the best CBD oil, CBD-rich flower, edibles, and more at dispensaries or delivery services, but make sure they are licensed and work with compliant partners who test their products based on state regulations.

✳ Generally, people are starting off with 5 to 30 milligrams of CBD per day for everyday relief. For more serious chronic health conditions, studies have shown that 5 to 25 milligrams of CBD per kilogram of body weight can deliver impactful results. Depending on how much you weigh, this could be an extremely high dose. There still isn't enough evidence to make a conclusion on what dosage is best, so if you are planning to take CBD at high doses, always be sure to consult with your health care professional to talk through application methods to avoid any risks.

✳ Taking higher doses of CBD does not mean it's the most effective way to use cannabidiol. The more CBD you consume, the greater the cumulative effect it has over time due to CBD's 24-hour half-life when taken orally. While you might not feel 5 milligrams of CBD per day at first, over a few weeks your CBD milligram intake will add up, potentially delivering longer-lasting effects. For best results, use a delivery method with high bioavailability rates and stick to a CBD regimen that works for you, even if it's a microdose of 1 to 2 milligrams per day. Start low, go slow.

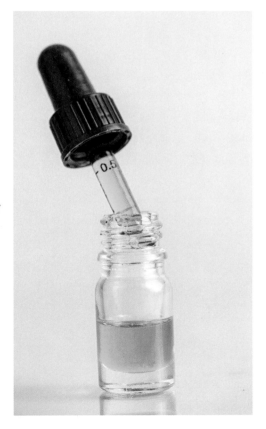

THE HIGH ART OF MICRODOSING

featuring Marcia Gagliardi, low-dose cannabis expert & founder of mymilligram

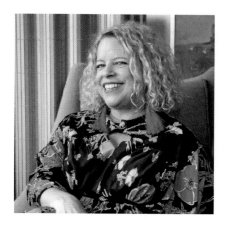

Marcia Gagliardi is a San Francisco–based culinary personality and writer, known for her tablehopper e-column about the SF dining scene. Her latest venture is her microdoser media brand, mymilligram. Her weekly newsletter (at mymilligram.com) is a resource for people who want to explore the intersection of cannabis and wellness in a low and slow way. Marcia writes in-depth features about low-dose, high-quality cannabis products made in California (with recommendations on how to carefully consume them) and she hosts educational events. Follow Marcia @mymilligram.

Marcia Gagliardi: "Microdosing is a hot topic, but before you announce you're a microdoser, you should clarify what it is you're microdosing because the term has its origins in the psychedelic world where it refers to microdosing LSD and psilocybin. I always clarify I'm talking about microdosing cannabis.

Cannabis is potent medicine, and can be highly effective and therapeutic, even at low doses (sometimes a low dose can actually be more effective than a larger one). You don't have to consume much to experience the plant's many therapeutic benefits, from help with pain to anxiety to sleep.

Some are sensitive to THC, and find it gets them too lifted and even anxious. But at a lower dose, THC can actually help with anxiety. Add some CBD in the mix, and it's even more beneficial (the two work very well in concert together as CBD lessens the lifted effects of THC, and THC increases the efficacy of CBD).

The goal is to start low and go slow, exploring cannabis at a sub-psychoactive level, and carefully consuming a measured dose until you discover your optimal milligram number. You should also investigate your ideal route of administration, such as sublingual versus edible—each route has a different onset time, effects, and duration.

(continued)

Typically, people experience effects from THC around 2 to 2.5 milligrams, although some require a higher dose to feel anything. Everyone has their own unique number. If you consume THC as an edible, expect the onset to take longer, and to potentially feel greater effects because THC is converted into a more potent form of THC when metabolized in the liver. It will also last longer, which can be a positive benefit. For this reason, I recommend trying to find your optimal number sublingually first, whether with a tincture or spray or tablet—it will be more consistent (what's in your stomach doesn't matter) and the effects should be more manageable. CBD doesn't have intoxicating effects, although people can experience calm, or energy, or even happy feelings from it, as well as diminished pain.

If you're exploring THC, I recommend starting with a balanced 1:1 tincture (1 part CBD, 1 part THC), as that way you get all the benefits from both cannabinoids. Start with 2 milligrams under your tongue. See how it feels (give it at least 45 minutes)—was it too much? Try less next time. Not sure? Try again the next day. Maintain for two to three days in a row, note any effects. You can then titrate up as needed, maybe try 2.5 milligrams for a few days, then 3 milligrams. Maybe go back to 2.5 milligrams. The goal is to find your perfect cruising altitude.

As for CBD, it's a trickier thing to microdose since the effects can be more difficult to notice in the beginning, but as one friend puts it: 'I definitely notice the days when I don't take CBD.'

Microdosing CBD allows you to explore relief from pain, anxiety, inflammation, and more, but be patient: it can take more than a month to start feeling the effects from a steady CBD regimen. If you're trying to discover the right dose for you, a good place to start is with 1 milligram of CBD for every 10 pounds (4.5 kg) of body weight. (You could even do half in the morning and half in the afternoon.) Remember that less is more, so start low and titrate up as needed after two weeks.

If you take other medications, it's always recommended to talk with your health care professional first."

HOW TO CHOOSE A TRUSTWORTHY BRAND

CBD has quickly become very popular. Unfortunately, due to a lack of regulations, there are more and more companies rushing to release items without going through proper safety checks and lab testing to ensure their products are up to par. Learning how to choose a trustworthy brand is crucial. By following the steps below, you will learn how to avoid marketing schemes and instead find the best, clean forms of CBD, THC, and any plant-based compounds. Treat your body like a temple; don't be afraid to ask the tough questions if something doesn't feel right.

KNOW YOUR PRODUCT FROM SOIL TO BOTTLE

To receive the best benefits from cannabis or hemp, you must find a reliable resource. It's extremely important to know where your product comes from because all cannabis- and hemp-based products are not created equal! If you're using hemp, look for products that are made from small production, organic therapeutic hemp farms. The ways in which large industrial hemp farms extract and manufacture cannabidiol typically do not make their products the best resources. Before purchasing, do your research and look into where the company is purchasing their cannabis and hemp from. If you cannot find this information online, reach out to the company to better understand how/where their products are made. If a company refuses to give you information, that's a big red flag.

THIRD-PARTY TESTING

As cannabis legalization continues, cannabis companies are working diligently to pass new state testing standards, ensuring that only the purest products will make their way to licensed dispensaries. Any quality brand should have lab results that they can share with you. Another step of quality assurance is third-party certification, such as TraceTrust, that ensures excellence in manufacturing processes, consumer safety, and product consistency. TraceTrust's "A True Dose," certification program ensures dose accuracy in legal cannabis and CBD ingestible products. The most trusted brands that go through this step are the companies that you can count on. Be aware that, as of now, there are no officially regulated testing standards in place for hemp CBD products. That said, if a hemp company has third-party testing results, this is a good sign that they are a reliable brand that cares about what they're producing.

FIND A DEPENDABLE MARKETPLACE

The last step to finding a reliable product is to look for a quality marketplace that vets their selection. A good example of this would be Eaze, where they stand behind every product that they put on their menu.

WORKING WITH CBD OIL

As you continue reading this book, you will discover that professionally made CBD oil products are extremely versatile and easy to work with. If you find a brand that you love, you can easily integrate it into your favorite beauty products, beverages, food recipes, and more as long as you use an *unflavored* item that won't conflict with the other ingredients you are working with.

If you do not intend to create your own CBD products at home (see chapter 2), select a reliable CBD oil that will be your companion for the recipes that are highlighted throughout each chapter. Every brand is different: Be sure to pay close attention to how many milligrams of CBD are in the oil you are working with.

Always estimate the dose per serving (i.e., how many milligrams per milliliter your product contains). Sometimes you have to calculate this information on your own, but don't fret! It's super easy. Simply divide total milligrams of CBD that's in the bottle by the total milliliters.

(Total Milligrams of CBD in Bottle) ÷ (Total Milliliters in Bottle) = Milligrams of CBD per milliliter

Once you perform this calculation, you can then gauge how many milligrams you'd like to include in the recipes based on your personal needs.

Please note: Each recipe contains a target dose based on *homemade* CBD items that contain varying levels of both CBD and THC, as well as an alternate recommendation for CBD-only dosing. However, feel free to customize your dose based on the item you are working with. Just be sure to estimate the final milligrams of CBD (or THC) per serving. This is really important, especially if you are preparing CBD items for others. Be responsible!

Useful Equipment

As you begin to browse the recipes in this book, you'll notice each one calls for its own tools and ingredients. What follows are some pieces of equipment that you'll find helpful when preparing self-care products, beverages, cuisine, and more. If you don't have all of the items on this list, don't stress or run out to buy everything. Use what you have and improvise when necessary.

Kitchen Accessories and Tools

Amber glass bottles with black poly cone or
   dropper cap

Baking pan

Bar spoon

Blender or food processor

Candy or instant-read thermometer

Cheesecloth

Cocktail strainer

Digital scale

Doggie bone cookie cutter
   (2½ inch [6 cm] recommended)

Double jigger

Small fine-mesh strainer

Funnel

Glass syrup bottle with stainless steel
   pourer

Herb grinder

Mason jars

Measuring cups

Measuring spoons

Milk frother

Muddler

Parchment paper

Peeler

Popsicle molds (stainless steel preferred)

Porcelain ramekins (set of 4)

Rolling pin

Saucepans, varying sizes

Shaker tin

Slow cooker

Sous vide precision cooker

Spice grinder

Spice jars

Tin containers

Vacuum seal

Vacuum seal bags

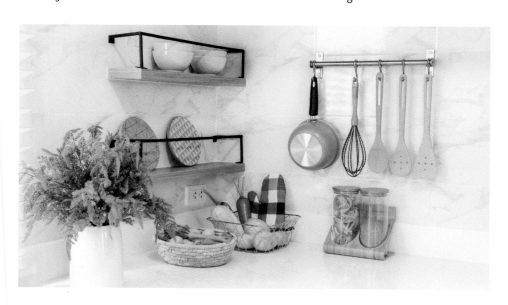

Products to Have on Hand

Below is a shopping list of the best products to line your kitchen cupboards with before making CBD infusions (see next chapter, page 51) and recipes. All of these items can be found at a licensed dispensary, online, or at your local health food store.

CBD Products

CBD-rich flower (best to purchase at a licensed dispensary)

   CBD-rich flower examples: ACDC, Cannatonic, Harle-Tsu, Critical Mass

CBD isolate powder (see Resources, page 206)

CBD cannabis oil or CBD hemp oil (start with your favorite *unflavored* brand)

Other Useful Products

Argan oil

Arnica oil

Beeswax pellets

Butter (European butter preferred)

Calendula oil

Chamomile oil

Coffee

Epsom salt

Essential oils (Purchase a kit so you can experiment with many different oils.)

Extracts, such as coconut, vanilla, and lemon, etc.

Flour

High-fat dairy or high-fat nondairy milks (e.g., cream, whole milk, coconut milk, or soymilk)

Honey (or other natural sweeteners, such as agave nectar)

Jojoba oil

Oat flower

Oat powder

Oils, such as MCT oil, olive oil, and coconut oil

Sparkling water

Sugar (both brown and granulated sugar)

Sunflower lecithin (both liquid and powder form)

Sweet almond oil

Terpene-rich fresh and dried herbs, such as mint, lavender, rosemary, thyme, and chamomile

Terpene-rich fruits, such as blackberries, strawberries, raspberries, blueberries, and lemon, etc.

Terpene-rich spices, such as cinnamon, turmeric, nutmeg, and cardamom, etc.

Vegetable glycerin

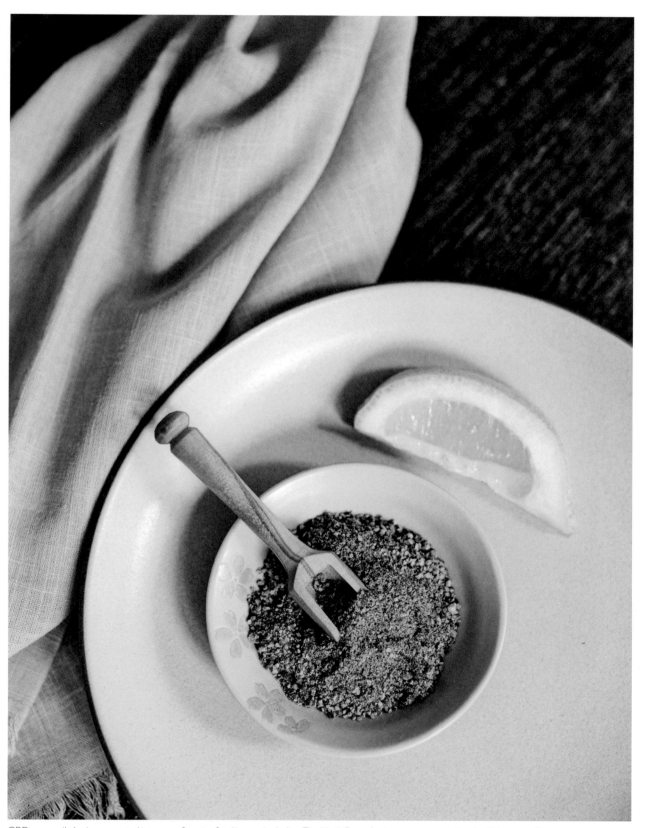

CBD can easily be incorporated into your favorite food items, including The Herb Somm's signature terpene-inspired Limonene Pepper.

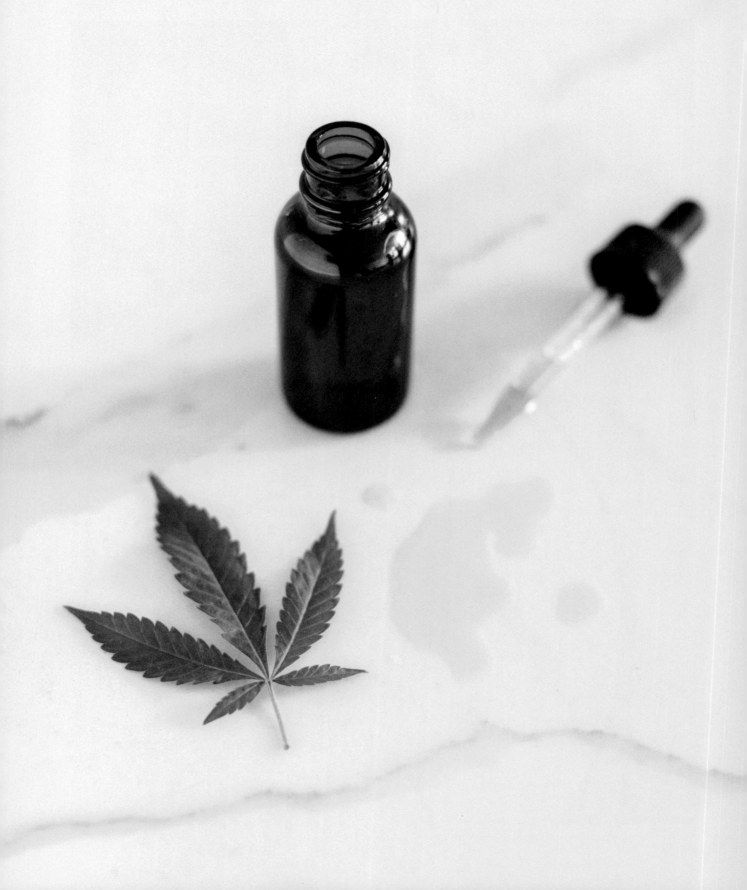

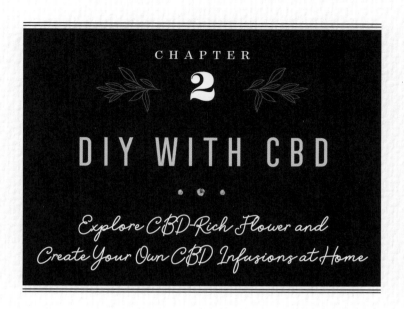

CHAPTER

2

DIY WITH CBD

• • •

Explore CBD-Rich Flower and
Create Your Own CBD Infusions at Home

I f you're looking to go the extra mile with CBD and learn how to craft your very own CBD oils, infusions, and tinctures, this chapter is for you. While professionally made products are the easiest first step for many beginners to experiment with, learning how to work with CBD-rich flower at home is a fantastic way to integrate natural healing compounds into your regimen. CBD is directly sourced from the cannabis plant, after all!

The best CBD medicine contains a full expression of cannabinoids and special molecules known as terpenes (page 44). By creating your own infusions at home, you have the ability to craft a product that best suits your personal needs. As long as you source clean, pesticide-free flower, you have the ability to customize a wide range of items, plus be in charge of quality control. You can rest assured that no dangerous fillers are in your CBD products, plus you won't have to worry about the fake or low-quality CBD oils that have flooded the market.

If you love DIY projects or simply enjoy learning new things, this chapter will provide you with the knowledge, tools, and techniques to easily work with cannabis or hemp flower. Explore the magical world of terpenes, learn how to interpret CBD:THC ratios, master decarboxylation, and create CBD oils, tinctures, butter, and more. Consider this your step-by-step guide in crafting CBD-rich products at home, which can later be used in the recipes throughout this book.

If DIY projects are not your thing or you don't have access to flower at this time, don't worry. Feel free to skip this chapter and use your professionally made CBD oil in the recipes. You can always come back if you're feeling adventurous!

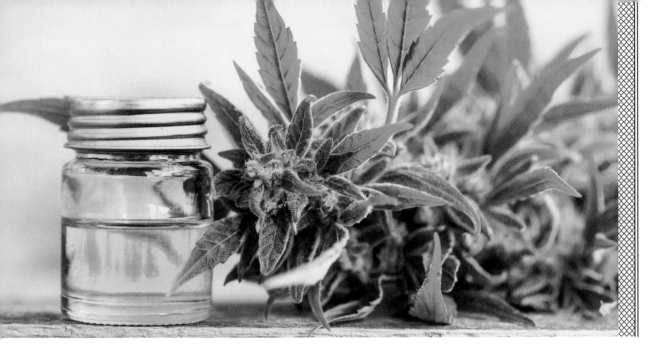

CBD-RICH FLOWER

The most effective CBD comes from high resin flower that contains a full expression of cannabinoids and terpenes. In this chapter, you will learn how to create your own CBD products using your choice of dried cannabis or hemp. Be aware that every strain is different, containing various ratios of CBD to THC. Though some strains have commonly reported anecdotal side effects, be aware that you might not feel the same way due to how your body processes phytocannabinoids and terpenes.

While there are hundreds of strains that contain varying levels of cannabidiol, there's a special select group known to be among some of the richest sources. Here are five strains that you should know.

ACDC

ACDC expresses high levels of CBD (around 20 percent CBD, 1 percent THC or 20:1 ratio). As a sativa-dominant phenotype of CBD-rich Cannatonic, ACDC is another powerful CBD-rich strain best known for its soothing abilities. It also reportedly works particularly well as a pain reliever as well as for anti-inflammatory, anti-nausea, and anti-anxiety applications. Because THC levels are so low, there are minimal intoxicating effects, making ACDC a great option for helping those who are seeking relief without getting high. Many have reported that they feel focused, happy, social, and relaxed while enjoying this strain. Its pleasant sweet citrus, pine, and spice aromas with bountiful earthy flavors come from higher levels of the terpenes myrcene, alpha-Pinene, limonene, and beta-Caryophyllene.

Cannatonic

This popular hybrid contains between 6 percent to 10 percent CBD and 3 percent to 17 percent THC, making it a more balanced strain. Cannatonic was born from a cross of

MK Ultra with G-13 Haze. It is renowned for its anti-inflammatory, antidepressant, and pain-relieving capabilities and might also aid those who suffer from migraines and insomnia. When consuming Cannatonic, you could feel incredibly relaxed with subtle euphoria. Similar to ACDC, Cannatonic has recognizable earthy and spice aromas and flavors due to myrcene and beta-Caryophyllene with hints of pine and citrus. You might also perceive soft floral aromas due to low levels of the terpene linalool.

Charlotte's Web

Perhaps one of the most famous CBD-rich strains is Charlotte's Web, developed for a five-year-old child, Charlotte Figi, who suffers from Dravet syndrome, which causes intense seizures. Because of the strain's high CBD potency ranging between 15 percent to 17 percent, and very low levels of THC, less than 0.3 percent, Charlotte's Web is considered to be a variation of hemp with little to no intoxicating effects. This hybrid strain is best known to help seizure disorders as well as provide relief for pain, headaches, and muscle spasms. After consuming Charlotte's Web, you might feel incredibly relaxed and mellow, while your palate is enticed with aromas and flavors of pine and earth with citrus and a soft hint of sage. Charlotte's Web is rich with the terpene myrcene.

Harlequin

Also displaying high levels of myrcene, Harlequin presents aromas and flavors of mango, citrus, and earth. Bred from Columbian Gold, Nepali indica, and Thai and Swiss landrace sativa strains (a.k.a. native strains), Harlequin is a wonderful option for pain relief as well as a possible solution for anxiety, depending on your internal chemistry. Because of its high levels of CBD, reaching as high as 15 percent, this sativa-dominant strain has been known to counteract THC's unpleasant paranoia side effects leaving you feeling only mild euphoria and blissful. Despite its relaxing side effects, Harlequin might also leave you feeling alert and focused, which could be in part due to its high levels of the terpene alpha-Pinene.

Harle-Tsu

For the CBD-rich flower recipes that are highlighted in this book, I used Harle-Tsu because of the high CBD to low THC ratio, which has been reported at 15 percent CBD to 1 percent THC before decarboxylation. As a cross between CBD-rich Harlequin and Sour Tsunami, Harle-Tsu might be a great option for managing chronic pain, inflammation, stress, and sleep disorders. The flavors and aromas are rounded out by notes of sweet citrus, pine, spice, and forest floor. A perfect option for anytime use!

Other CBD-Rich Strains

To further explore CBD-rich strains, look for Sour Tsunami, Haleigh's Hope, Ringo's Gift, Dancehall, Suzy Q, Omrita Rx, Valentine X, Critical Mass, and Canna-Tsu.

THE MAGICAL WORLD OF TERPENES

One of the building blocks and most crucial compounds that differentiates plants and herbs are terpenes. Terpenes are the organic compounds that give cannabis all of the wonderful aromas and flavors that you can perceive when smelling your favorite strains. Unlike CBD, THC, and the other phytocannabinoids that are just found in cannabis, terpenes are found in many different fruits, vegetables, herbs, spices, and botanicals. You can think of terpenes as the spice of life! More than 200 terpenes have been identified in cannabis so far, each with varying aroma and flavor profiles as well as unique therapeutic properties. Here is a quick look at six common terpenes along with their distinctive characteristics.

ALPHA-PINENE

Alpha-Pinene, also known as α-Pinene, is a principal monoterpene that is beneficial for plants, animals, and humans. This important compound is found in pine trees and other conifers, but high levels of alpha-Pinene can also be found in cannabis, pine needles, pine nuts, dill, rosemary, and other herbs. Much like walking through a forest, this refreshing terpene has the ability to help with asthma, acts as an anti-inflammatory, provides energy, promotes alertness, and can aid in memory retention.

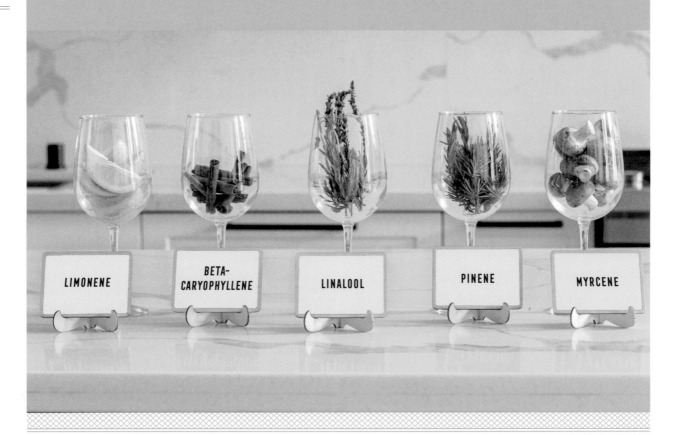

LIMONENE

BETA-CARYOPHYLLENE

LINALOOL

PINENE

MYRCENE

BETA-CARYOPHYLLENE

Beta-Caryophyllene, also written as β-Caryophyllene, is a therapeutic terpene that is characterized by its spicy black pepper, cinnamon, and clove notes. It is known to be a natural pain reliever, reduces inflammation, and acts as an antioxidant, and it protects the brain, nervous system, and body by binding to CB2 receptors. It is also one of the most prevalent terpenes found in cannabis.

LIMONENE

Limonene is the citrusy terpene that displays strong lemon, lime, grapefruit, and tangerine characteristics. Not only is this terpene beneficial for aromatherapy purposes, it is also a natural stress reducer, can enhance moods, promotes weight loss, and fights depression. Limonene is also often added to medical ointments and creams to help penetrate the skin.

LINALOOL

Lavender is the first thing that comes to mind when thinking of linalool. This restorative terpene is responsible for the memorable fragrance of this calming purple flower as well as other florals including citrus blossoms, violets, and roses. Linalool promotes relaxation and sleep, as well as a sense of well-being and is used in many essential oils, soaps, and bath and body products. Linalool is known to have blissful side effects.

MYRCENE

Myrcene, or β-Myrcene, is known to be one of the most common terpenes found in cannabis. This comes as no surprise as hundreds of cannabis strains display myrcene's signature funky notes of mixed herbs, forest floor, mushroom, skunk, tropical fruits, and earthy undertones. A few well-known CBD strains that contain pronounced levels include Cannatonic, Harlequin, and Harle-Tsu. As a natural remedy, studies have shown this terpene has the ability to relax muscles, slow bacterial growth, promote sleep, and can help with diabetes.

NEROLIDOL

Nerolidol is a useful terpene that is found in several strains of cannabis. It has multiple therapeutic uses, but is also well known for killing things that can harm plants, animals, and humans. This includes bacteria, fungi, parasites, spider mites, etc. Despite its heroic qualities, humans can safely ingest it and inhale it without any issues. Nerolidol is also easily absorbed through skin, which makes it an excellent addition to CBD topicals, such as lotions, moisturizers, and salves. It is also a common ingredient that's found in perfumes as it has a pleasant scent that can be described as perfumey and floral-like jasmine with slight hints of wood and ginger flower.

UNDERSTANDING CBD:THC RATIOS

featuring Elise McRoberts, cannabis educator, thought leader & event producer

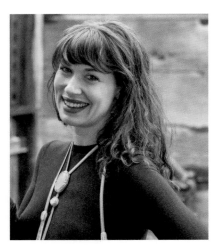

Elise McRoberts is an entrepreneur, producer, and public personality focused on elevating the cannabis space through education, community, and culture. One of the early outspoken advocates of microdosing and using cannabis for everyday wellness, Elise judged her first Cannabis Cup for High Times magazine in 2012 and began working with California brands in 2013. An effective consultant in business development, brand strategy, and communications, Elise established herself as a top advisor to cannabis brands, as well as a trusted expert to a fan base of cannabis enthusiasts and canna-curious followers on social media. Follow Elise @elisemcroberts.

Elise McRoberts: "Broadly speaking, there are three types of ratio-based cannabis products that you might come across. They are:

Type 1 (THC-dominant)—famously intoxicating cannabis varietals
High THC, low CBD cannabis is known for miracle stories such as shrinking cancer tumors. Example: Rick Simpson Oil.

Type 2 (THC & CBD)—intoxicating, but not as edgy as THC-dominant varietals
Mixed THC and CBD cannabis is the most common and used for everything from daily wellness, to depression and anxiety, to chronic pain and autoimmune disorders.

Type 3 (CBD-dominant)—nonintoxicating cannabis or hemp
High CBD, low THC strains are used in places where cannabis-derived CBD is still prohibited, and often on children and those unable to tolerate any amount of THC.

Understanding CBD-to-THC ratios is just like knowing how fractions work. For instance, 1:1 or 4:1 would look like ⅟₁ or ⁴⁄₁ as a fraction that represents the amount of CBD to THC, usually in milligrams.

The industry standard is to list ratios as CBD to THC; this is how it will appear on most product labels. But if you're ever worried, just read the label carefully and it should be clear. A 1:1 (pronounced "one to one") product means the makeup is 1 part CBD equal to 1 part THC, whereas a 4:1 (pronounced "four to one"), would equate to 4 parts CBD to 1 part THC.

While products vary, you still need to know your dose with ratios, so be sure to read all label information on the product before using and begin with a low dose or the dose that is recommended by the brand.

A good place to start might be an 18:1 tincture (18 milligrams of CBD for every 1 milligram of THC). Start with a quarter of a dropper, which would equal around 4.5 milligrams of CBD to 0.25 milligrams of THC. How do you feel? Based on the results, you can go up or down in milligrams until you find a perfect balance, but remember to be patient. If you don't feel effects right away, adjust the dosage the next time you decide to use the product.

Another technique that you might try is choosing a high CBD-to-THC ratio for daytime usage to help with more minimal aliments, and then increase the THC for nighttime usage to help with sleep or if you're not feeling enough relief. The most common ratios are: 20:1, 18:1, 4:1, 3:1, and 1:1.

I consider 1:1 the perfect miracle daily vitamin, which, in low doses, seems to benefit many people from chronic pain to anxiety. Research is also showing that greater amounts of CBD can actually decrease or neutralize the THC high, depending on the amount of each compound that is present in a particular product. Thus, a greater ratio of CBD-to-THC means feeling less high.

Remember, cannabis affects everyone differently. While some people might experience results with very little THC, others might need a higher dose. As of now, the only way to discover your perfect ratio is by experimentation.

When you try different ratios, always be sure that you experiment with products *within the same brand*. Just as unique as the cannabis plant is, there are also hundreds of variations on extraction method and production, therefore, an 18:1 by one brand is not equal to an 18:1 by another brand. I highly recommend Care By Design as a starter brand. Their website is also a great resource for ratio information as well as other informative websites such as ProjectCBD.org.

Above all, there are no right or wrong answers when it comes to discovering your perfect ratio. Choose a brand that you love, explore a few of their ratio options, and enjoy the journey."

DECARBOXYLATION & INFUSIONS

Throughout this book, you will encounter recipes that you can experiment with at home including infused beverages, cuisine, beauty products, pet treats, and more. Most of these recipes can be made with store-bought CBD products (page 35). However, because I believe that using clean, pesticide-free CBD-rich cannabis flower provides the greatest benefits, most of them can also be made using handcrafted infusions that you can make yourself.

Before you attempt to do any of these things, there are some important concepts that you must learn when it comes to working with cannabis and hemp products, including an introduction to decarboxylation and infusions.

DECARBOXYLATION

To unlock the ultimate healing elements of CBD and THC, you must decarboxylate your dry cannabis flower before integrating it into a recipe. Decarboxylation is a heating process that triggers the chemical reaction that releases the carboxylic acids from CBD and THC to fully activate cannabis. In other words, you are converting CBDA to CBD and THCA to THC.

While there are many approaches to decarboxylation, the method that I've found most success with exposes dry cannabis to heat between 240°F and 295°F (115°C–146°C) for 20 to 60 minutes. Heat for a shorter time at higher temperatures or for a longer time at lower temperatures between this range. For example, if you're using a higher temperature (between 275°F and 295°F [135°C–146°C]), bake for 20 minutes max and be careful not to overcook. Overheating can degrade cannabinoids and terpenes!

For the purposes of this book, you are going to use a decarboxylation technique that I learned from professional cannabis chef Coreen Carroll of the Cannaisseur Series. To do so properly, pre-heat your oven to 275°F (135°C). As your oven is heating, line a baking sheet with aluminum foil or parchment paper. Begin to break up the dry flower into pea-sized pieces with your fingers or scissors and spread the cannabis evenly onto your baking sheet. Once the oven is heated, simply put the baking sheet in the oven and bake for 20 minutes. Remove from heat, let cool, and store in an airtight sealed mason jar until you're ready to infuse it into a recipe. See more from Chef Coreen Carroll on page 164.

If you're planning to make a variety of recipes, you can decarboxylate large batches of flower and save portions of it for future use. Please note that if you use the oven method to decarboxylate, your kitchen will fill with very potent cannabis aromas, so if you're worried about attracting unwanted attention from your neighbors, it might be best to use another method such as sous vide (page 154) or a decarboxylation device (page 50).

Regardless of what method you choose, as you're decarboxylating, do not exceed 300°F (150°C) at any time—the hotter you heat the cannabis, the more likely it is that you'll diminish the precious cannabinoids and terpenes that are there. Turn to page 55 to learn more about activation temperatures and boiling points.

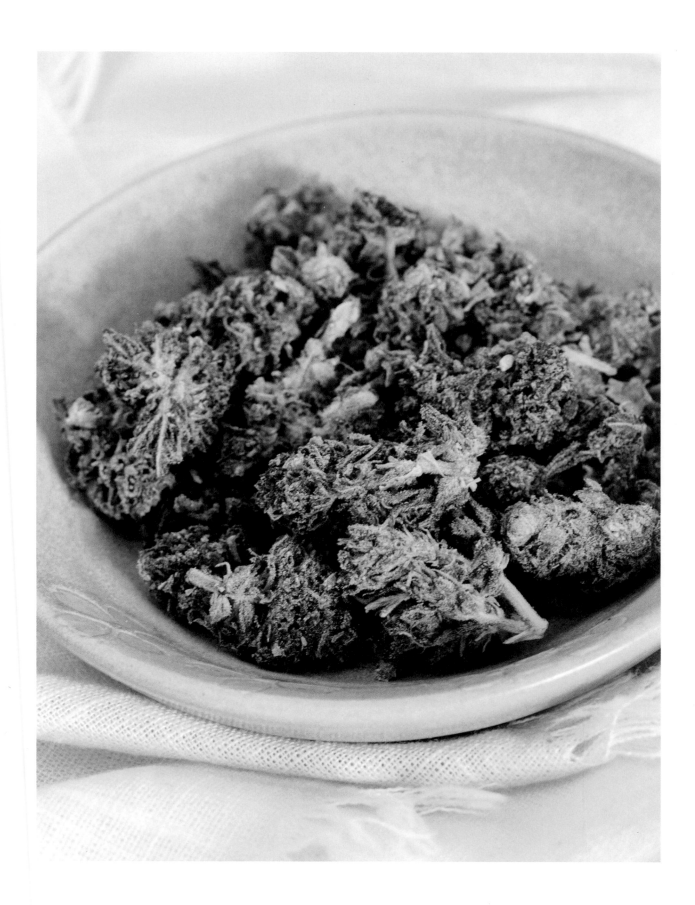

EXPLORING DECARBOXYLATION AND INFUSION DEVICES

If you're someone who loves the idea of easy cooking or simple infusions with the click of a button, a decarboxylation or infusion device might be the tool for you. Below is a list of some of the best devices available at the time of writing.

LEVO INFUSION DEVICE

LEVO's infusion device is designed exclusively for infusing botanicals into oil and butter. The company's LEVO II device also comes with decarboxylation capabilities, which makes the process of cooking with cannabis or hemp that much easier. If you're tech savvy and looking for a device that can decarb and make infusions well, LEVO is for you. Visit www.levooil.com.

ARDENT NOVA DECARBOXYLATOR

If you're looking for a consistent decarboxylation method, the Ardent NOVA decarboxylator is a fantastic tool as it provides a perfect combination of time and temperature that fully activates your flower. The company has also created an infusion sleeve that you can put into the device to create your very own infused oil, butter, caramels, and more. This is a great option for any beginner! Visit www.ardentcannabis.com

THE MAGICALBUTTER MACHINE

The MagicalButter machine has become a cult favorite among professional and at-home chefs alike. This easy-to-use device was designed specifically for one purpose: to create recipes and botanical infusions with little to no effort. This device is great for those who are looking to make a variety of infusions including butter, oil, lotions, and more. Visit www.magicalbutter.com

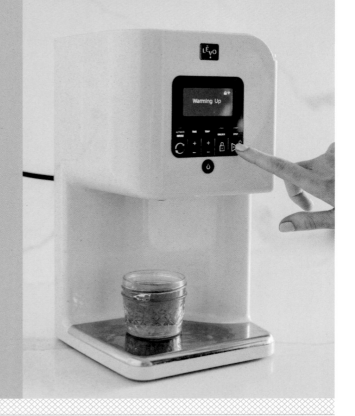

INFUSIONS

Creating an infusion is one of the best ways to integrate CBD into food, drinks, self-care products, and more. We'll be using the technique for extracting chemical compounds (cannabinoids, terpenes, etc.), from cannabis or therapeutic hemp using an alcohol-based or fat-based solvent such as olive oil, coconut oil, or butter. Both CBD and THC are especially drawn to fats, making them lipophilic or fat-soluble compounds. This means they break down or dissolve in fats or lipids, which is why you see many oil-based cannabis and hemp products on the market. Some of the most common carrier oils that you'll come across include MCT oil, olive oil, hemp seed oil, and grape-seed oil.

To create your own infusions at home, there are many methods that you can use including the stovetop method, a slow cooker, sous vide (page 154), or an infusion device (see opposite). There are pros and cons to each method, but for the purposes of this book, you will mostly use the stovetop method as it is fast, efficient, and easy, plus you'll most likely already own the equipment that's needed (i.e., a stovetop, saucepan, Mason jars, and candy or instant-read thermometer). The only downsides to this method are inconsistent heating and having to keep a close eye on the infusion until it's done cooking. That said, if you can use the sous vide method, this is a terrific way to make infusions, especially if you're trying to preserve terpene profiles. Turn to page 154 for Monica Lo's signature "Sous Weed" method.

To practice making CBD-rich flower infusions at home, flip to the end of this chapter to create a CBD Olive Oil (page 61), CBD Coconut Oil (page 63), and CBD Butter (page 64).

DOSING CALCULATIONS

Learning how to calculate dosages for the products you are making at home is very important, especially if you're working with THC. Keep in mind that using a professionally made oil or isolate in your recipes is very straightforward and easy to accurately dose. If you're making a dry flower infusion, it's difficult to precisely measure the strength of your infusions without the help of a potency checking tool. That said, by learning how to calculate an estimate of how much CBD or THC is in your infusions, you can avoid the pitfalls. Follow this strategy for best results.

KEY THINGS TO REMEMBER WHEN MAKING DRY FLOWER INFUSIONS

To estimate the total amount of CBD and THC that will be in your infusion, you must combine CBD + CBDA and THC + THCA percentages to determine the potency. This information should be listed on the packaging of the flower when you purchase it.

Multiply the CBDA or THCA by a 0.877 conversion rate and add it to your CBD and THC to get your total CBD and total THC. If CBDA and THCA percentages are not listed on the packaging, then this conversion has most likely already been done for you.

THE DOSAGE CALCULATION

This formula can be used to calculate the final amount of CBD and THC per serving, based on various infusion bases.

Step 1: Determine how much total CBD or THC is in your dry flower after you purchase it.

Example: For the recipes in this book, I used Harle-Tsu that measured at a total of 15 percent CBD and 1 percent THC before decarboxylation.

0.53 (CBD) + [16.25 (CBDA) * 0.877] = 14.78 or 15% Total CBD

0.05 (THC) + [0.90 (THCA) * 0.877] = 0.8393 or 1% Total THC

Step 2: Convert CBD and THC percentages to determine milligrams per gram of dry flower (1 gram = 1,000 milligrams).

Example: Based on the starting values in Step 1, 15 percent CBD and 1 percent THC

0.15 x 1,000 mg/g = 150 mg CBD per gram of dry flower

0.01 x 1,000 mg/g = 10 mg THC per gram of dry flower

Step 3: After you decarboxylate the flower, account for loss during the heating process if you're using an oven. (33 percent estimated when using a standard oven to decarb).

Example: Remaining after 33 percent loss

150 mg/g x 0.67 = 100.5 mg/g CBD

10 mg/g x 0.67 = 6.7 mg/g THC

Step 4: Multiply the remaining CBD and THC from Step 3 by grams of flower called for in your recipe.

Example: For butter, the recipe calls for 3.5 grams of CBD-rich flower

100.5 mg/g x 3.5 grams = 351.75 mg CBD

6.7 mg/g x 3.5 grams = 23.45 mg THC

Step 5: Convert your primary infusion ingredients (i.e., olive oil, butter, coconut oil, etc.) into grams.

To make the conversions easy, here is a quick conversion guide that lists some of the ingredients that you'll use in this book.

Example: 1 cup butter = 227 grams

INGREDIENT	SERVING SIZE	GRAMS
Coconut Oil & MCT Oil	1 cup	216
Olive Oil	1 cup	219
Butter	1 cup	227
Water	1 cup	240
Milk	1 cup	255

Step 6: When heating your flower infusions for longer periods of time, you must account for loss due to evaporation. Use the chart below to calculate the remaining volume of your ingredient after loss.

After you account for the percentage loss, you have your final yield:

227 grams of butter x 0.75 = 170.25 grams (final yield)

INGREDIENT	% LOSS OF VOLUME DURING INFUSION PROCESS
Oil	20% (Heating 2–3 Hours)
Butter	25% (Heating 2–3 Hours)
Water (Simple Syrup)	12.5% (Heating 1 Hour)
Milk	12.5% (Heating 1 Hour)

Step 7: Determine the number of servings remaining in your final yield. Divide your answer from Step 6 by the number of grams per serving, indicated in the chart below.

Example: Based on the yield above

170.25 grams / (14.18 grams of butter per tablespoon) = 12 tablespoons of butter or ¾ cup as indicated in the recipe on page 64)

INGREDIENT	SERVING SIZE	GRAMS
Oil (olive, coconut)	1 tablespoon	13.75
Butter	1 tablespoon	14.18
Milk	1 ounce	28
Agave Nectar Simple Syrup	1 ounce	28
MCT Oil Tincture	1 milliliter	0.95

Step 8: Finally, Divide Your Remaining CBD and THC from Step 4 by the number of servings in Step 7. This gives you CBD and THC per serving.

Example: Final calculation for butter

351.75 mg / 12 tablespoons = 29.3 or 29 mg CBD per tablespoon

23.5 mg / 12 tablespoons = 1.9 or 2 mg THC per tablespoon

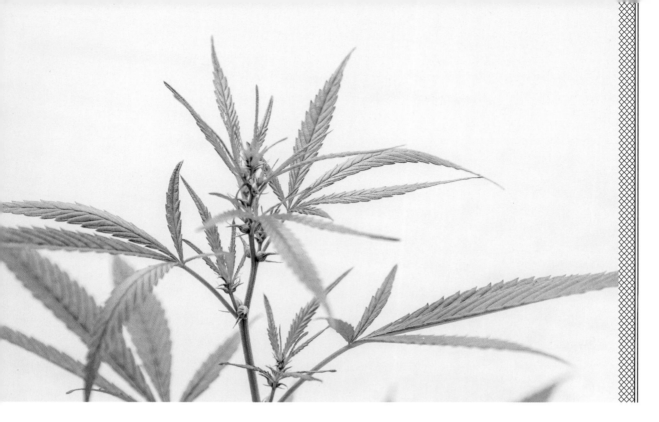

ACTIVATING CBD & THC, PLUS OTHER IMPORTANT BOILING POINTS

There's an art to cooking with cannabis. While it might seem like you're heading back to chemistry class, don't stress. All you need to know are the activation temperatures and boiling points of a few chemical compounds before you start creating recipes. These particular temperatures are also needed to allow other compounds to become available to ensure that you are getting the most effectiveness out of your products.

Although CBDA and THCA are the primary phytocannabinoids you'll want to activate via decarboxylation, each phytocannabinoid and terpene has their own unique boiling points when heated. If you exceed these temperatures, the compounds will begin to degrade resulting in loss. This is something you want to avoid to receive the best end results.

Remember, if you're using a professionally made CBD or THC product, there is no need to activate the item unless directed.

Select a decarboxylation method that works best for you (refer back to page 48) and use the following guide as you begin cooking with herbal products.

PHYTOCANNABINOID & TERPENE DECARBOXYLATION TEMPERATURES AND BOILING POINT GUIDE

Activation Temperatures for Decarboxylation

PHYTOCANNABINOIDS	F°	C°
THCA*	240°–275°	115°–135°
CBDA**	240°–295°	115°–146°

*Converts from THCA to THC if you heat between 240°F and 275°F (115°C–135°C) for 20 minutes to 1 hour

**Converts from CBDA to CBD if you heat between 240°F and 295°F (115°C–146°C) for 20 minutes to 1 hour

Boiling Points

Stay below these temperatures to avoid the degradation of these precious compounds

PHYTOCANNABINOIDS	F°	C°
CBG	248°	120°
THC	314°	157°
CBD	320°–356°	160°–180°
CBDv	356°	180°
CBN	365°	185°
THCv	428°	220°
CBC	428°	220°

TERPENES	F°	C°
Nerolidol	252°	122°
beta-Caryophyllene	266°	130°
alpha-Pinene	311°	155°
Myrcene	334°	168°
Limonene	349°	176°
Terpinolene	366°	186°
Linalool	388°	198°

MASTERING CBD TINCTURES

featuring Gillian Levy, president & co-founder of Humboldt Apothecary

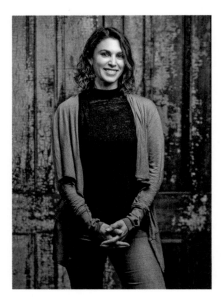

Gillian Levy is the president and co-founder of Humboldt Apothecary, a women-owned cannabis tincture company in the heart of Humboldt County. She is also a botanist, herbalist, cannabis advocate, and mother of two teens. Gillian and her business partner, Susan Cleverdon, created Humboldt Apothecary with a vision of crafting cannabis-based products that could target and support healing and wellness for a variety of conditions. Gillian and Susan have used their love and knowledge of medicinal herbs to formulate blends of plants that synergize well with cannabis to create maximum therapeutic benefits. The company has a commitment to using only the highest quality, most environmentally sustainable ingredients, and that includes 100 percent sun-grown cannabis from Humboldt County. Follow Gillian @HumboldtApothecary or visit www.humboldtapothecary.com.

Gillian Levy: "Before making your first CBD tincture there are a few important things that every beginner should know. First off, CBD goes well in many different applications and is a powerful medicine. Because of its ability to balance the functions of the endocannabinoid system, it is responsible for modulating almost every physiological system in our bodies. This means CBD tinctures can be very effective for treating a variety of conditions. If you're thinking of making tinctures at home, here are a few things to keep in mind:

Making a basic cannabis tincture can be extremely simple and anyone can do it with a few basic tools.

A true tincture, by definition, is in an alcohol base. However, there are a variety of liquids that can be used to create a DIY tincture. I recommend using alcohol, as well as oils such as olive- or coconut-derived MCT oil.

Tinctures are desirable because they have a long shelf life. They are also a healthy alternative to sugar-laden edibles and can be incorporated into your daily routine in a convenient and discreet manner.

If you are making a cannabis tincture, you will want to make sure that you are using an appropriate liquid for extraction. For example, glycerin is not a very effective solvent for extracting cannabinoids. Instead, I would recommend using an oil or alcohol for making high-quality tinctures.

In order to achieve best results, I prefer to use only whole-plant extracts that contain a suite of different cannabinoids, including THC and CBD. Because CBD and THC are most commonly found together in the cannabis plant, I don't tend to focus on one or the other for combining with other botanicals. I don't work with isolates; however, depending on what your needs are, both CBD and THC have their specific indications. In general, most people can tolerate CBD more readily—it is something that can be incorporated into a wellness program throughout the day.

While most people find that using a pure THC formula during the day is not suitable if they need to function at work, etc., there are some that find that THC is the perfect constituent to calm the mind and promote focus. That said, everyone responds differently to CBD and THC. When creating a tincture, it is best to determine your ideal ratio of CBD:THC versus just choosing either CBD or THC.

Whether you are using a manufactured tincture or a homemade tincture, the beauty of these products is convenience. I like to carry a tincture with me so that I can take it when needed. In general, I will take my oil-based tinctures sublingually and I will take my alcohol tinctures in a bit of water or tea. It is ideal to consume a tincture with a little food that contains some fat content, because that is the most efficient way to maximize absorption of the cannabinoids. If I have a little more time on my hands, I really enjoy creating mocktails with tinctures as an elegant and tasty alternative to an alcoholic drink."

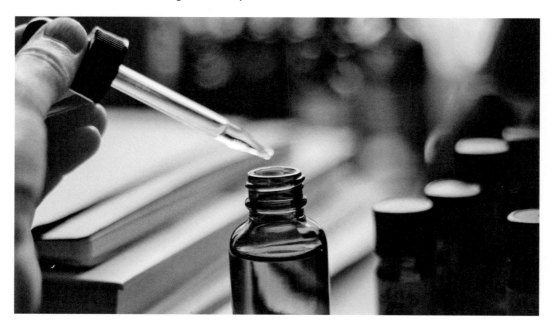

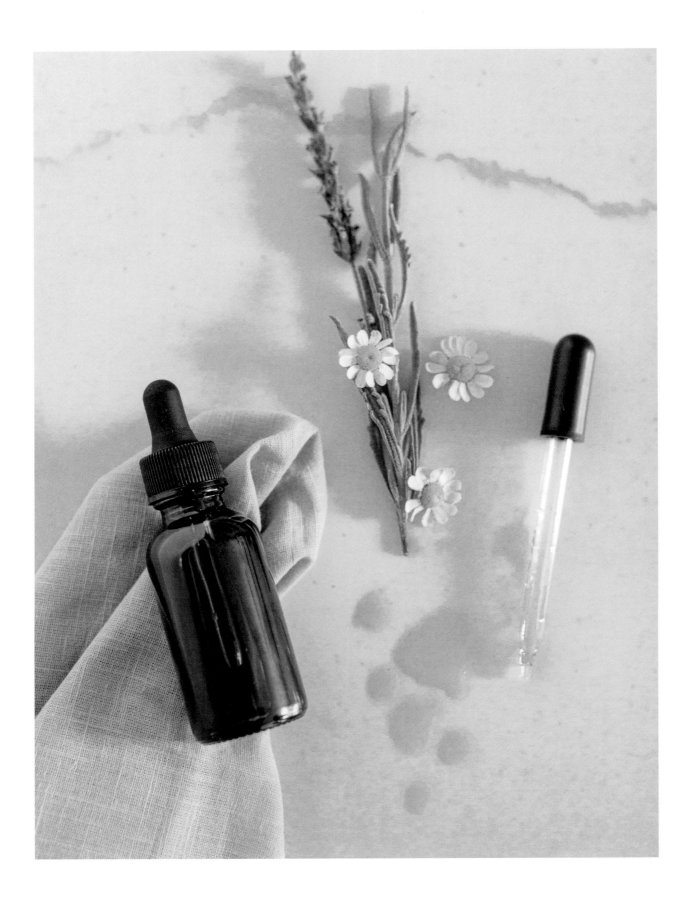

BEST SLEEP EVER CBD OIL TINCTURE

Now that you know the basics when it comes to CBD tinctures, it's time to make your own. To get your toes wet, one of the simplest beginner recipes is to create a CBD oil tincture at home.

One of the primary reasons I love using cannabis products is that they can help promote a good night's rest. To establish a healthy sleep routine, practice the same wind-down rituals night after night to signal to your brain that it's time for rest. CBD can become a part of that bedtime ritual. Try making this CBD tincture for your best sleep ever!

YIELD: 4½ ounces (135 ml)

TARGET DOSE: 5 mg CBD | 0.3 mg THC per ml
(see pages 31 and 36 for more on dosing calculations)

EQUIPMENT
Digital scale
Two 8-ounce (240-ml) sterilized
    Mason jars
Measuring cup
Small saucepan
Thermometer
Oven mitt
Cheesecloth
Fine-mesh strainer
Amber glass bottle with dropper cap
Funnel

**7 grams decarboxylated CBD-rich
    flower (page 42)**

2 tablespoons (5 g) dried lavender

1 tablespoon (1 g) dried chamomile

½ teaspoon dried valerian root

½ teaspoon dried passion flower

**¾ cup (177 ml) MCT oil or fractioned
    coconut oil**

Weigh out 7 grams of CBD-rich decarboxylated cannabis flower. In a Mason jar, combine the cannabis, lavender, chamomile, valerian root, passion flower, and MCT oil. Seal the top tightly.

Fill the bottom of a small saucepan with water, making sure to allow enough space so that the water will not hit the top of the Mason jar. Set the Mason jar inside and begin to heat on low. Continue to heat over a gentle boil (around 200°F [93°C]) for 2 hours, making sure the water does not exceed 211°F (99°C). Check in frequently and refill the saucepan with water as needed due to evaporation. When finished, remove the Mason jar safely with an oven mitt and let the jar cool.

Prepare the cheesecloth by placing it over the fine-mesh strainer. Pour the infused MCT oil over the cheesecloth into a clean Mason jar. Gently press (but do not wring out) to extract the oil. Once the mixture has cooled, transfer your CBD oil mixture into an amber glass bottle using a funnel and secure with a dropper cap.

Store at room temperature in a dark cabinet to best preserve and shake well before using.

NOTE

This recipe can also be made using high-proof Everclear. Simply mix the cannabis and ingredients with high-proof alcohol in your Mason jar. Close the jar and place the mixture in a cool, dark place. Let it sit for about 2 to 3 weeks, agitating the Mason jar every so often. Once ready, use cheesecloth and a fine-mesh strainer to filter out the herbs, and place the tincture into a dropper bottle for easy use. To store properly, keep your CBD tincture in a cool, dark place. Never heat!

MASTERING CBD INFUSIONS

Before you start making the more complicated recipes found in this book, you'll need to create CBD olive oil, CBD coconut oil, and CBD butter infusions using CBD-rich flower. I used Harle-Tsu flower that measured at a total of 15 percent CBD and 1 percent THC before decarboxylation.

Remember, your numbers will differ depending on the strain and source that you use, so be sure to calculate your own CBD/THC milligrams per serving before making your infusion (refer back to page 52 for at-home dosage calculations). Do your best to make an accurate estimate, and always conservatively sample each batch before serving to others. After you create these essential ingredients, on to the other recipes in the next chapters!

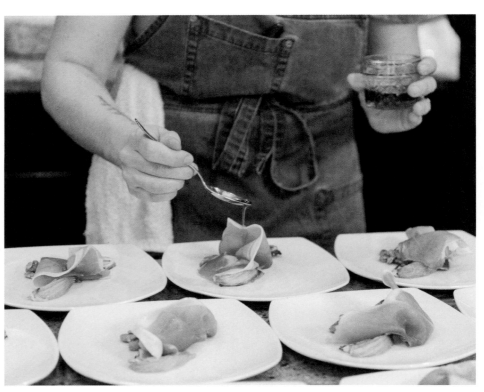

Chef Coreen Carroll adds CBD-infused olive oil to cuisine at The Herb Somm's Feast of the Flowers event in San Francisco.

CBD OLIVE OIL

Creating infused olive oil is an essential ingredient for any at-home chef looking to make elevated cuisine. By mixing CBD olive oil into a variety of recipes, you can easily infuse just about anything. Here's how to create a CBD olive oil at home using CBD-rich flower.

YIELD: ¾ cup (175 ml)	TARGET DOSE: 1 tablespoon = 28 mg CBD | 2 mg THC

EQUIPMENT

Digital scale

One 16-ounce (480-ml) sterilized
    Mason jar

Measuring cup

Small saucepan

Thermometer

Oven mitt

Cheesecloth

Fine-mesh strainer

One 8-ounce (240-ml) sterilized
    Mason jar

**3.5 grams CBD-rich decarboxylated
    cannabis flower**

1 cup (236 ml) olive oil

Weigh out 3.5 grams of CBD-rich decarboxylated flower. In a 16-ounce (480-ml) Mason jar, combine the cannabis flower and olive oil. Seal the top tightly.

In a small saucepan, fill the bottom of the pan with water, making sure to allow enough space so that the water will not hit the top of the Mason jar. Set the Mason jar inside and begin to heat on low. Continue to heat over a gentle boil (around 200°F [93°C]) for 3 hours, making sure the water does not exceed 211°F (99°C). Check in frequently and refill the saucepan with water as needed due to evaporation. When finished, remove the Mason jar safely with an oven mitt and let the jar cool.

Prepare the cheesecloth by placing it over the fine-mesh strainer. Begin to pour the infused olive oil over the cheesecloth into a clean 8-ounce (240-ml) Mason jar. Gently press (but do not wring out) to extract the oil. Avoid squeezing the cheesecloth because this will extract unattractive chlorophyll flavors.

Store at room temperature in a dark cabinet to best preserve.

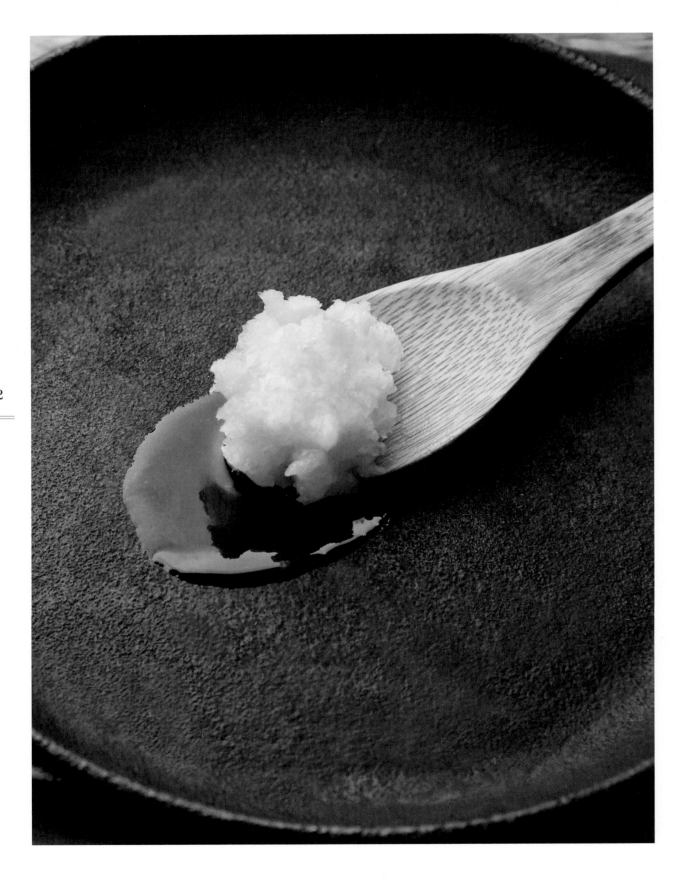

CBD COCONUT OIL

Much like olive oil, coconut oil is an incredibly versatile ingredient that can be used in a variety of recipes, particularly desserts and self-care products. The process for CBD-infused olive oil and for infusing CBD coconut oil is almost the same; the only difference is the addition of water to help purify and clarify your CBD coconut oil.

YIELD: ¾ cup (164 g)	TARGET DOSE: 1 tablespoon = 28 mg CBD | 2 mg THC

EQUIPMENT

Digital scale

Measuring cup

Two 16-ounce (480-ml) sterilized
    Mason jars

Small saucepan

Cheesecloth

Fine-mesh strainer

Oven mitt

Thermometer

**3.5 grams CBD-rich decarboxylated
cannabis flower**

1 cup (218 g or 240 ml) coconut oil

1 cup (240 ml) water

Weigh out 3.5 grams of CBD-rich decarboxylated cannabis flower. If you're using unrefined coconut oil that's hardened, make sure to melt it down to measure exactly 1 cup (240 ml). In a Mason jar, combine the cannabis flower, coconut oil, and water. Seal the top tightly.

In a small saucepan, fill the bottom of the pan with water, making sure to allow enough space so that the water will not hit the top of the Mason jar. Set the Mason jar inside and begin to heat on low. Continue to heat over a gentle boil (around 200°F [93°C]) for 3 hours, making sure the water does not exceed 211°F (99°C). Check in frequently and refill the pan with water as needed due to evaporation. When finished, remove the Mason jar safely with an oven mitt and let the jar cool.

Prepare the cheesecloth by placing it over the fine-mesh strainer. Pour the infused coconut oil over the cheesecloth into a clean Mason jar. Refrigerate overnight to separate the water.

The next day, use a knife to loosen the sides of the CBD coconut oil that's hardened in the top of your Mason jar. You can either poke a hole through the side and drain out the water or use a spoon to transfer the oil to a smaller clean container and then drain the water.

To store, seal in an airtight container, label, and keep in the refrigerator for best results.

NOTE

Throughout this book, CBD-infused fractionated coconut oil or MCT oil might be called for in a recipe. Fractionated coconut oil is different than coconut oil because it does not solidify at room temperature—it is always in liquid form, which makes it a perfect ingredient to combine with an Epsom salt soak or massage oil (see pages 95 and 98, respectively). To make your own at home, simply follow the instructions for making a CBD-infused olive oil on page 61, but use fractionated coconut or MCT oil as your base ingredient instead of olive oil (do not add water).

CBD BUTTER, TWO WAYS

If you love cooking, then you already know that butter is a staple ingredient to have in your kitchen when preparing recipes. By using a similar method to infusing coconut oil, you can easily create CBD butter by using a slow cooker or the stovetop method. CBD butter can be stored in the freezer for basically forever (okay, maybe more like a year), but be sure to defrost it overnight in the refrigerator before using. Here are two ways to make CBD butter using CBD-rich flower and CBD isolate.

CBD-RICH FLOWER BUTTER

YIELD: ¾ cup (168 g)	TARGET DOSE: 1 tablespoon = 29 mg CBD | 2 mg THC

EQUIPMENT
Digital scale
Two 16-ounce (480-ml) sterilized
   Mason jars
Measuring cup
Medium saucepan
Thermometer
Oven mitt
Cheesecloth
Fine-mesh strainer

**3.5 grams CBD-Rich decarboxylated
   cannabis flower**
1 cup (225 g) butter (2 sticks)
1 cup (240 ml) water

Weigh out 3.5 grams of CBD-rich decarboxylated cannabis flower. Cut the butter into cubes. In a Mason jar, combine the butter, cannabis flower, and water. Be sure to put the butter on the bottom of the jar so it melts first. Seal the top tightly.

In a medium-sized saucepan, fill the bottom of the pan with water, making sure to allow enough space so that the water will not hit the top of the Mason jar. Set the Mason jar inside and begin to heat on low. Continue to heat over a gentle boil (around 200°F [93°C]) for 3 hours, making sure the water does not exceed 211°F (99°C). Check in frequently and refill the pan with water as needed due to evaporation. Agitate the jar every now and then using an oven mitt. When finished, remove the Mason jar safely with an oven mitt and let the jar cool.

Prepare the cheesecloth by placing it over the fine-mesh strainer. Pour the infused butter over the cheesecloth into a clean Mason jar. Gently press to extract the butter; do not squeeze the cheesecloth because this will extract unattractive chlorophyll flavors. Refrigerate overnight to separate the water.

The next day, use a knife the loosen the sides of the CBD butter that's hardened at the top of your Mason jar. You can either poke a hole through the side and drain out the water or use a spoon to transfer the butter over to a clean container and then drain the water.

To store, seal in an airtight container, label, and then place it in the refrigerator or freezer to best preserve.

CBD ISOLATE BUTTER

YIELD: **1** cup (225 g)	**TARGET DOSE:** 1 tablespoon = 30 mg CBD

EQUIPMENT

One 16-ounce (480-ml) sterilized
   Mason jar
Small saucepan
Thermometer
Measuring spoons
Oven mitt
One 8-ounce (240-ml) sterilized
   Mason jar (optional)

1 cup (225 g) butter (2 sticks)

**0.48 grams CBD isolate powder
(480 mg CBD)**

Cut the butter into cubes and add it to a 16-ounce (480-ml) Mason jar. Fill a small saucepan with water, making sure to allow enough space so that the water will not hit the top of the Mason jar.

Set the Mason jar inside unsealed and begin to heat on low heat until it reaches 140°F to 150°F (60°C to 66°C). The butter should melt at this point, but be careful that the water around the Mason jar never reaches a boil.

Add the CBD isolate powder. Begin to stir the mixture and continue to heat for another 5 to 10 minutes, or until the CBD isolate is completely integrated. Remove from the heat using an oven mitt and transfer it to a smaller 8-ounce (240-ml) Mason jar if you wish. Give the butter a few good stirs.

To store, seal in an airtight container, label, and then place it in the refrigerator or freezer to best preserve.

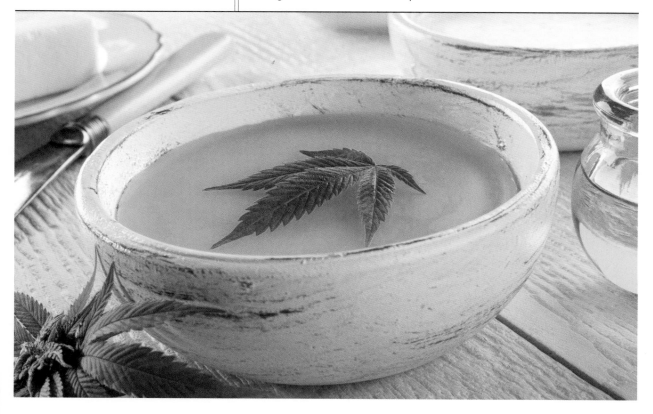

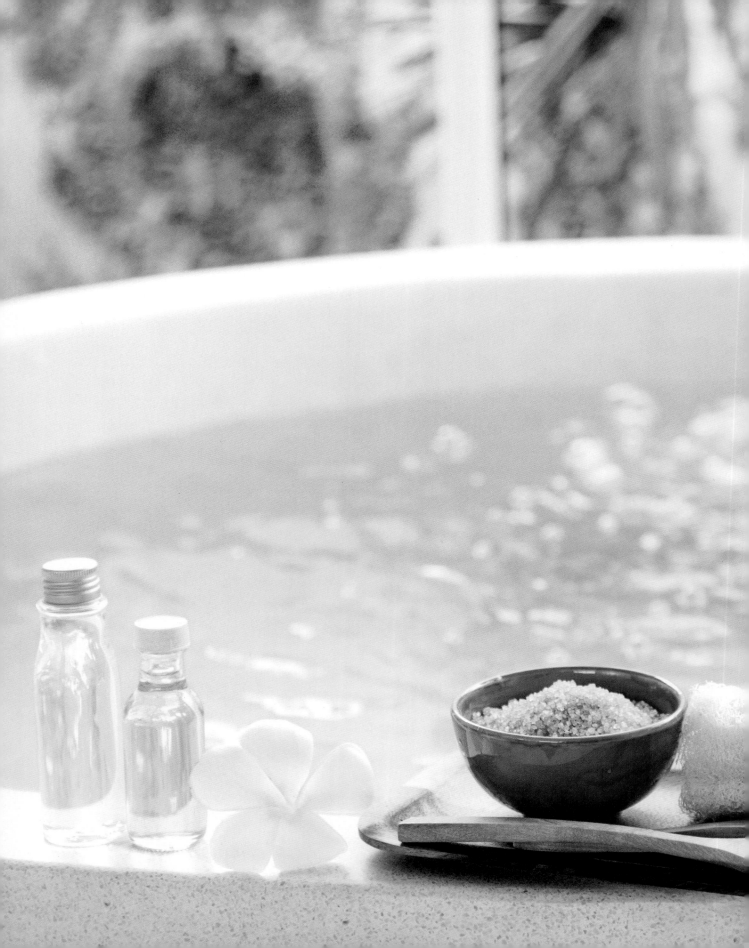

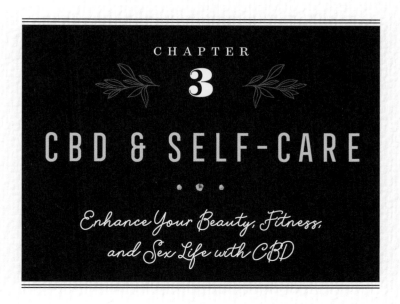

CHAPTER

3

CBD & SELF-CARE

Enhance Your Beauty, Fitness, and Sex Life with CBD

Self-care is the ultimate practice that can benefit your life, your relationships, and your overall happiness. Hitting the pause button and dedicating a few hours a week to "me time" is necessary to maintain homeostasis.

CBD-rich products can be tremendous tools that you can use in your own self-care regimen. Whether using a tincture, bath bomb, or soothing CBD salve, if done with intention, CBD can work with our bodies to comfort the mind, body, and spirit.

Whether you are looking to incorporate CBD into your beauty or fitness routine, or to get intimate with a partner, the coming pages will cover a wide range of self-care topics. Learn the tips and tricks on how to create nourishing products at home. Relax, take a deep breath, and find your inner Zen with CBD. I hope you're ready to take your self-care regimen to the next level.

SELF-CARE 101

It's easy to get caught up in the daily grind and hustle, leaving self-care as the lowest priority on your task list. Even though it might seem like your to-dos are never-ending, be sure to carve out time for rest and relaxation—*take care of yourself*. Here are four simple ways to incorporate CBD in wellness routines to promote a happier, healthier life.

1. Establish a healthy skin care routine.

Establishing a healthy skin care routine is one of the easiest things you can do to improve your self-care. Repeat after me: cleanse, tone, moisturize. While this ritual might sound obvious to most, you'd be surprised by how many people skip this basic and essential self-care practice, particularly men. The great news is there are some incredible new CBD skin care products available that will help boost your personal hygiene. Skip to page 73 to learn more about the benefits of using CBD for skin care and discover products that might be right for you.

2. Start your day with gentle stretching or meditation.

One of the best ways to start the day is with a few simple calming activities such as stretching or meditation. One way to incorporate CBD into this regimen is to use topical products. For stretching, simply apply a salve or lotion to the target area of your stretch. For an at-home meditation, turn to page 81 for some calming words to follow by Dee Dussault, founder of Ganja Yoga.

3. Stay on top of your fitness routine.

With an overly demanding schedule, fitness routines can often sit on the back-burner. While many of us have intentions to finally hit the gym or that new fitness class, life can get in the way, distracting us from much-needed exercise time. Setting aside just 30 minutes of physical activity a day can improve your daily routine, leaving you feeling more present and in tune with yourself. CBD is a powerful tool that you can incorporate into your fitness regimen. See page 78 for some tips on how CBD can enhance your workout routine.

4. Get intimate.

Getting intimate with your partner is a fantastic way to boost your self-care. Not only can sex (or self-pleasure) relieve stress, but it can help you sleep better, act as a form of exercise, and is a bonding experience. Did you know you can use CBD to enhance those intimate times? Yes, it's true. Turn to page 83 to learn more.

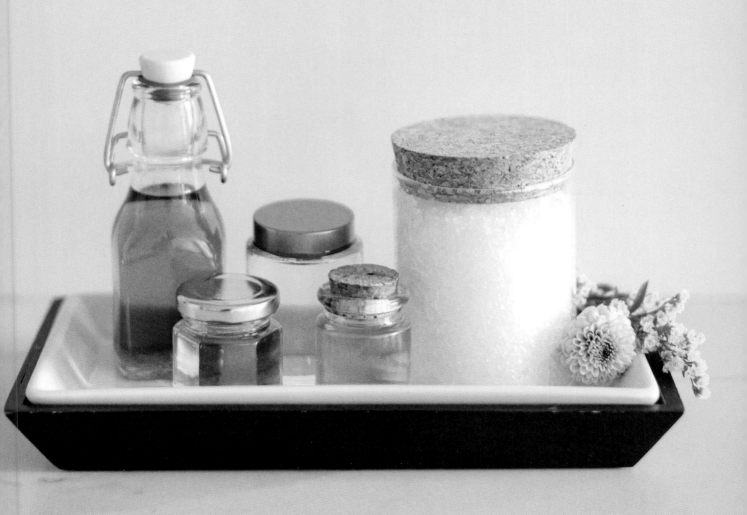

SECRETS TO OPTIMIZING CBD FOR SELF-CARE

featuring Kimberly Dillon, founder of Plant and Prosper & Frigg Wellness

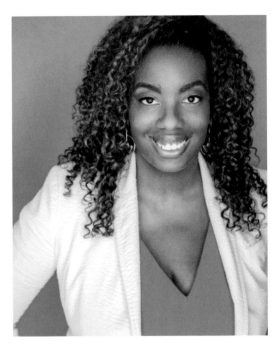

Kimberly is the founder of a cannabis strategy consultancy, Plant and Prosper, where she speaks on the topics of Cannabis & Women's Health and CBD & Self-Care at conferences such as Goop, Adweek, and SXSW. She is also the founder of Frigg Wellness, a product line tackling the impacts of stress head on. In 2018, Adweek named her one of LA's Brand Stars. As the former Chief Marketing Officer for Papa & Barkley, Kimberly helped position the brand as the number-one selling cannabis topical and tincture brand in California. She currently lives in Los Angeles, and in addition to her work with Plant and Prosper, she also performs stand-up comedy. Follow Kimberly @kimberlykdillon.

Kimberly Dillon: "We live in a world of stress. There are so many things out of our control like the political landscape, climate change, rising housing costs, and underemployment. It is easy to get overwhelmed. Making space for yourself is important for both your mental and physical well-being. If you drive your car too long in the hot desert, there is a chance that it will overheat and you will have to pull over and let the engine cool down. Like cars, humans can also overheat and burn out. The goal should be to avoid that state. I think of self-care as preventive medicine. I use CBD and other plants proactively, so I won't burn out from stress.

My self-care routine begins in the morning. I add full-spectrum CBD powder to my coffee or smoothie. It's part of my morning ritual and it allows me to feel balanced for the rest of the day. I also like to apply CBD oil all over my face and body. I have found that CBD facial serum has cleared my skin and has faded some of my fine lines. When I have massages, I also ask my massage therapist to use a CBD body oil. You have not lived until you've added CBD into your bodywork!

My advice to beginners is to understand the science behind what you are buying and using to understand how the products will work. CBD is definitely not one size fits all, and that mentality can be dangerous—so take the time to explore what works for you.

When it comes to whole-plant products, you should also be aware that pricing is not standardized. Ideally, you should be paying for the amount of active ingredient in the product. That said, compare milligrams of CBD to cost to calculate the cost per milligram. You want your money to go to milligrams of CBD, not filler materials like oil. I believe CBD can be a guidepost for other industries like beauty, especially with active ingredient transparency and product testing. As consumers, we should know how much of each active ingredient is in the product, how and where these ingredients are sourced, and know that those ingredients are clean and free of metals, pesticides, and microbials.

We are just in the beginning phases of CBD products. In the near future, stay tuned for big things in skin care, haircare, and food!"

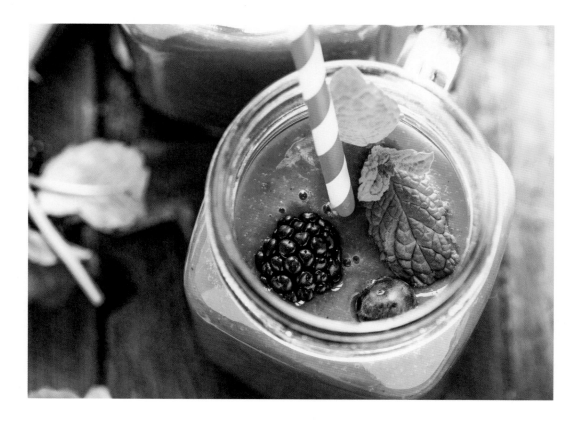

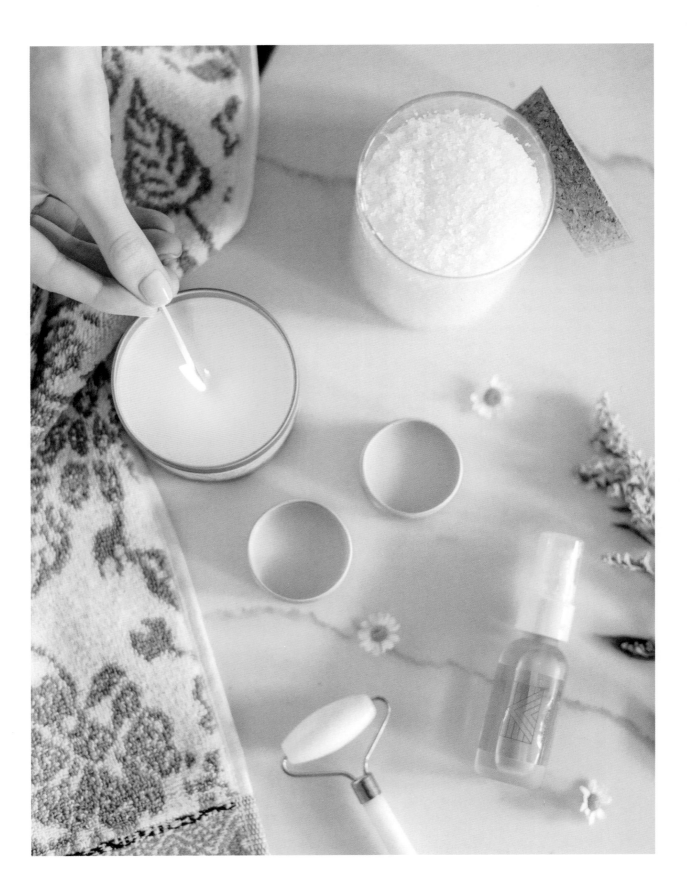

CBD & SKIN CARE

CBD is quickly becoming a popular ingredient for skin care products. While cannabidiol is making an appearance in just about every beauty item these days, you might be wondering how CBD impacts your skin and what are its benefits?

It turns out that this up-and-coming beauty ingredient is packed with antioxidants and powerful anti-inflammatory properties that can benefit the skin, particularly with redness, puffiness, swelling, and soreness, which are common side effects of some of the most challenging skin conditions. CBD is a beneficial ingredient because it absorbs quickly into the skin, which is why it's often added to lotions, face oils, lip balms, salves, and creams. Because of these conditions, it's naturally suitable to be used as a wholesome beauty product ingredient.

There are hundreds, if not thousands, of beauty products currently on the market that contain harsh, unrecognizable ingredients that are not good for your skin. In comparison, most of the high-quality CBD skin care products contain limited ingredients and are sourced from all-natural materials. Look for full-spectrum CBD items to ensure your skin receives the ensemble of other important cannabinoids and terpenes that supercharge CBD's healing benefits.

If you suffer from acne, CBD might also help treat this condition due to its anti-inflammatory properties and ability to reduce sebum production in the skin, which causes outbreaks. Studies have also shown that CBD can help prevent and disrupt the activation of pro-acne agents like inflammatory cytokines, which can make the problem worse. This is great news for those who are seeking acne solutions in addition to making skin appear more radiant and youthful.

CBD is still a newcomer in the beauty world. Compared to skin care power players such as retinol, research on CBD is still in its early stages, but you can rest assured it is showing potential as an active ingredient that can help with varying skin needs.

THC skin care products and topicals can reduce inflammation as well, but they also have the enhanced ability to relax muscle spasms and offer a better solution for pain relief. Products containing THC can help with facial tension, headaches, sore jaw muscles, and more. While both THC and CBD have analgesic and anti-inflammatory properties, when comparing the two, you can consider THC a better solution for pain relief whereas CBD is likely to be the better anti-inflammatory.

NOTE

THC skin care products are generally not intoxicating so you will not feel high after using them; however, there are a few exceptions. Infused bath bombs, Epsom salt soaks, and transdermal patches containing THC can enter your bloodstream, although you will not feel the same "high" effects as you would after eating an edible or smoking a joint. In the coming pages, you will learn more about these applications in greater detail.

CBD BEAUTY PRODUCTS & HOW TO USE THEM

Now that you know the benefits of CBD skin care, you're probably wondering what products are best to use. Just like any other CBD item, the source of your CBD skin care product matters. Not all CBD is created equal. If you're looking for the real deal, do not get hemp seed oil confused with hemp-derived CBD oil. It's not the same!

You should also be aware of dosing. As of now, there are no standards for how much CBD should go into beauty products, so total milligrams per product varies across the board. The source of your CBD is what matters the most, so don't think a higher potency means a higher-quality product. Be smart, read labels, and do your research.

Here is a list of some of the most popular CBD beauty products that are currently available online or in your favorite retail stores. Have fun exploring one or all of these exciting categories!

CBD Bath Bombs & Epsom Salt Soaks

CBD bath bombs and Epsom salt soaks are easy products to incorporate into your self-care routine. The best products contain all-natural ingredients and 100 percent organic essential oils to calm and rejuvenate the body. For bath bombs, simply fill your bathtub with the water temperature of your choice, drop the bath bomb in, and soak. Allow yourself at least 30 minutes to fully soak in the CBD and essential oils. For Epsom salt soaks, rub the Epsom salt and CBD oil into your skin first, and then add the rest of the contents into warm water as directed and soak your body for at least 30 minutes. Both of these products can also be used as part of your fitness regimen, particularly Epsom salt soaks. Epsom salt contains magnesium sulfate, which helps promote muscle relaxation. As your body rests in the warm water, CBD and magnesium sulfate team up to release waste that has built up after vigorous exercise.

Keep in mind that both of these bath items can also be infused with THC. If you use one, THC can enter the bloodstream through your colon as you soak. While you probably won't feel the same high as you do with oral consumption methods, bath bombs and Epsom salt soaks can offer some mild euphoric effects. See page 95 for a CBD Rosemary Blossom Epsom Salt Soak recipe.

CBD Body Scrubs

Do you have rough patches of skin that could use some exfoliation? CBD body scrubs can nourish dry skin and gently exfoliate dead skin cells, leaving your skin glowing. To use, apply the CBD body scrub in the bath, shower, or for a self-pedicure. When applying, be careful *not* to saturate the CBD scrub with water. Rub the scrub onto target areas or your full body. Once the desired exfoliation is achieved, rinse with warm water and follow up with CBD lotion to soothe the skin.

CBD Body Butter & Lotions

CBD body butter and lotions are meant for maximum coverage. You don't need to rinse them off and the CBD can rest on your skin: this allows your skin to absorb the healing molecules. CBD body butter tends to be a thicker cream, whereas CBD lotion is more lightweight. To use, simply massage the lotion or body butter onto your skin, allowing it to fully absorb. This process will not only nourish the skin, but it should also ease minor discomfort and help with inflammation.

CBD Facial Serums, Masks & Oils

The three most common CBD facial treatments include serums, masks, and oils. CBD facial serums tend to be the thinnest products, so they should be the first thing that you layer onto your skin after washing and toning. To use, apply the serum to clean skin and gently massage it in until it's absorbed. CBD facial masks are another option. If you have time during the day, you can apply it to your skin and leave it on as directed, or use an overnight CBD mask. Finally, CBD face oils are an option for those with drier skin. To use, apply three to five drops to cleansed and toned skin morning and night. For a Honey & Oat CBD Facial Mask, turn to page 91.

CBD Lip Balm

If you have dry, cracked lips, CBD lip balm is a must-have. When looking for a good lip care product, be sure to pay close attention to what other ingredients are in the balm. Coconut oil, shea butter, cacao butter, kokum butter, and jojoba oil are all nourishing ingredients that won't further dry out your lips. Avoid lip balms that contain hyaluronic acid and glycerin, ingredients that will actually make problems worse. Apply the CBD lip balm liberally to clean lips as needed using your clean fingertips. Repeat throughout the day. See page 92 for a CBD Coconut Chamomile Lip Balm.

CBD Roll-Ons

If you're on the go, try a CBD roll-on. They are compact and convenient, meant to alleviate stress when you're desperately in need. To use, apply to your temples, neck, forehead, sore jaw muscles, wrists, or pressure points. Massage the oil into the skin until it's absorbed.

WHAT YOU NEED TO KNOW ABOUT CBD BEAUTY PRODUCTS

featuring Claudia Mata, founder of Vertly

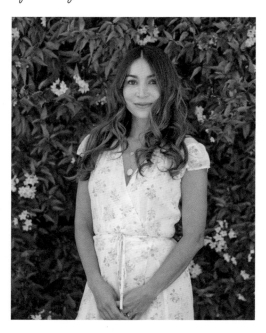

Claudia Mata is the founder of Vertly, a plant-based, clean beauty skin care line that focuses on the natural wellness properties of CBD. After relocating from New York City to the San Francisco Bay Area, Claudia immersed herself into a formal herbalism education, which she then merged with her husband's background in cannabis to create what is now Vertly. Prior to this, Claudia worked in fashion editorial in NYC for twelve years, most recently as the Accessories and Jewelry Director at W Magazine. Claudia is based in Northern California, where she lives with her husband and their two children. Follow Claudia @vertlybalm or visit www.vertlybalm.com.

Claudia Mata: "Vertly is a full-spectrum CBD and botanical-infused clean beauty and skin care line. Based in Northern California, we source locally grown herbs to create our potent herbal extractions in-house. Our approach is to harness botanical powers by combining CBD with other plants, which can be especially beneficial for the skin.

When people are thinking of incorporating our products, or cannabidiol in any form, into their skin care routine, there are three things I think every beginner should know:

1. CBD is derived from hemp or cannabis, and like many other healing plants with anti-inflammatory properties, it can be extremely beneficial in promoting skin wellness.

2. Look beyond the CBD. Having cannabinoids in your skin care routine is great, but it's important to ensure the other ingredients in your products are also clean and beneficial.

3. Be realistic with your expectations of CBD—it's not a magic bullet that will cure all, but it can help you feel better and relieve some skin inflammation.

I apply small amounts of CBD to be absorbed into the skin through daily use. I'm also a big advocate of microdosing—using approximately 1 to 2 millgrams of CBD per application on my face, focusing on overall skin wellness. It's equally important to pair this microdose of CBD with various other complementary anti-inflammatory plant extracts in order to enhance their benefits. Because CBD is fat soluble and can stay bound to your cells, you can build up a reserve and just use a smaller amount daily for maintenance. I use it for preventative measures, because inflammation can sneak up on even us healthy folks!

When purchasing a CBD beauty product, all of the ingredients in the product are just as important as the CBD. The way ingredients are grown and processed make a big difference, as does their freshness. Make sure you use products that source clean and therapeutic ingredients—it's being absorbed through your skin into your body!

Finally, it's important to experiment to find what dosage works for you: everyone will have their own unique needs and responses. We all have different levels of inflammation and absorption rates of cannabinoids that vary from person to person. What I love about plant medicine and plant healing is that it requires us to listen to our own body on what's working and what's needed as opposed to prescribing a specific amount of something for everyone across the board. That said, have fun experimenting with different full-spectrum products to see what works best for you."

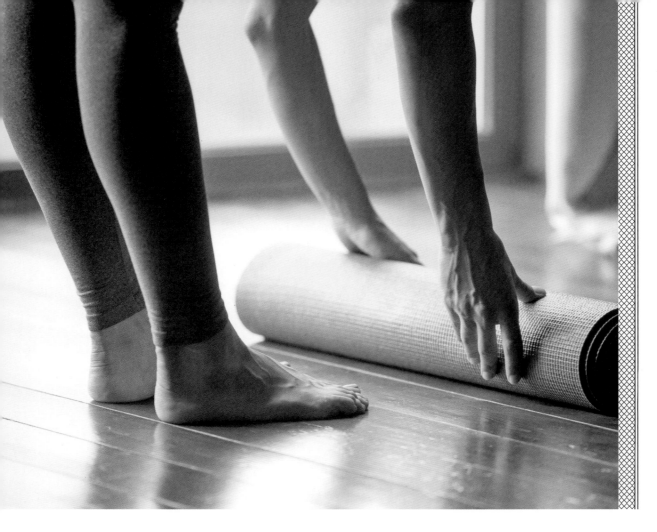

CBD & FITNESS

If you're an athlete or fitness junkie you might be wondering if CBD can enhance fitness routines. While it probably won't make you jump higher or run faster, some athletes are finding success by using it as a supplement and topical to help battle inflammation, reduce anxiety, and eliminate race-day jitters.

Depending on which consumption method you choose, there are various ways you can integrate CBD into your fitness routine. While some athletes prefer to use CBD the night before a big workout, others prefer to use it afterward to help with recovery.

Although there isn't conclusive research to support CBD's performance-enhancing abilities, there is an abundance of anecdotal evidence that suggests it can help athletic performance. For instance, one thing we do know is that CBD can help with inflammation and can reduce muscle spasms. Every time you exercise, your body experiences some wear and tear. While mild inflammation is necessary during the recovery process, too much can make things worse, causing more serious injuries. Keep in mind, taking multiple ibuprofens in a row to battle inflammation can actually have a negative impact on your kidneys. CBD might work for you as an alternative.

If you're an athlete who is drug tested frequently, you should avoid cannabis-derived CBD that contains higher levels of THC because the THC will show up. Instead, try broad-spectrum hemp-derived CBD. Get to know your product, look at the product's test results for cannabinoid percentages, and modify your dosages accordingly.

If you're dealing with an injury, CBD balms or salves might be a valuable tool to help with recovery. Because you can target the troubled area directly, these topicals have been known to help soothe sore muscles and reduce swelling; however, some athletes have reported that they've found the most success when using CBD to treat long-term trouble areas rather than sudden injuries.

If you decide to try CBD before you exercise, be sure to test the product first so there are no surprises later on. If you are comfortable with the results, start with a small serving using the application of your choice. Depending on what method you choose to use, it can take anywhere from 30 seconds if you vape up to 1 hour or more if you eat an edible for effects to kick in.

Remember, CBD is *very* subtle so you will not feel the head change or pronounced sense of euphoria that THC brings. For best results, if you are taking a sublingual, softgel, or edible, take it 1 to 1½ hours before exercising and be sure to drink plenty of water. Be aware that CBD can cause drowsiness for some people. This is why some athletes prefer to take it at night or use it for recovery instead of using directly before a big workout. Everyone is different, and it's best to establish your own CBD regimen that works for you.

A QUICK NOTE ABOUT THC

According to a *Journal of Science and Medicine in Sports* analysis, studies showed that THC does not enhance aerobic/cardio exercise or strength. Instead, these studies showed adverse side effects. However, this research was not conclusive to all forms of fitness. In some cases, THC can be a useful companion to some sports and can help athletes focus. It really depends on how your body reacts to THC. Dee Dussault, founder of Ganja Yoga, believes that cannabis and THC can deepen your yoga practice (see page 80).

HOW TO INCORPORATE CBD INTO YOUR YOGA PRACTICE

featuring Dee Dussault, founder of Ganja Yoga

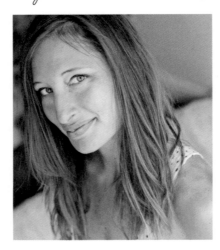

Dee Dussault is the first yoga teacher to publicly offer cannabis-enhanced yoga. Over the past decade, she's taught Ganja Yoga to thousands of students across the country. As a seasoned yoga practitioner of more than twenty-three years, Dee is also an international speaker and the author of the book Ganja Yoga *(HarperCollins). Her groundbreaking work has been featured in the* New York Times, Business Insider, Newsweek, *and many other national publications, and she's been featured in major international media from Japan to France. Follow Dee @GanjaYoga or visit deedussault.com.*

Dee Dussault: "For me, CBD is a daily supplement. I use it to relieve anxiety, pain, and stress. I recommend CBD to my yoga clients who are new to cannabis but want to benefit from its healing properties. I also offer it at every class in case someone over-consumes THC, as CBD can mitigate some of the paranoia that too much THC can bring. Because it's an anti-inflammatory agent and offers some pain relief, CBD can be used before yoga to help people get the gumption to do the yoga class. I think that's potent!

If you're thinking about using CBD in your yoga class, I would recommend you try CBD in topical form. If you choose to inhale isolated CBD, I'd recommend you supplement with small doses of THC (if you have access to it) to get the full range of the cannabinoids, terpenes, and other active ingredients. If you don't have access to THC products, hemp CBD is an alternative, but make sure it's organically grown.

Topicals are an ideal way to use cannabis and CBD because they get us practicing self-touch and self-massage, both of which are under-appreciated parts of daily life. To practice using CBD with yoga at home, here is a CBD topical meditation that you can try at home."

GANJA YOGA CBD TOPICAL MEDITATION

Using the CBD topical of your choice, start to rub it into any areas that express pain, tension, tightness, stiffness, or anywhere else that you feel needs work—begin to close your eyes. Shutting one sensory gate allows deeper feelings in the other senses. Breathe deeply. There's no rush, just *be here now*, and allow the passing of thoughts, feelings, and physical sensations. How little effort can you put into the massage, where you're not using energy, but getting it? Perhaps try rubbing the topical in, then use a massage ball to give the grunt work to an inanimate object. However you do it, use a deep, full exhale to relax even more fully. Enjoy as long as possible.

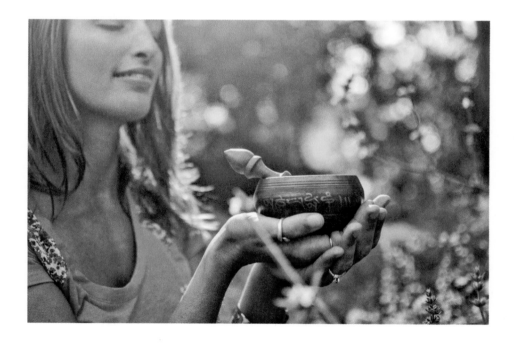

CBD FITNESS PRODUCTS & HOW TO USE THEM

Here is a list of some of the most popular CBD fitness products that athletes are finding success with. Depending on your body, metabolism, and what activity you are planning to do, effects can vary from person to person. The best part about CBD is that you won't get intoxicated from consuming too much, so don't be afraid to combine products from all categories (tinctures, edibles, topicals, etc.) as you figure out a CBD fitness regimen that works best for you.

CBD Balms & Salves

Topicals are a go-to during post-workout recovery because you can target problem areas directly. For example, if you are a runner and have sore feet after a long-distance run, CBD balms or salves make a perfect massage ointment to rub onto your feet to relax the muscles and soothe minor aches, pains, and chafing. When compared, CBD balms are typically firmer and will need to be massaged into the skin longer than a softer salve. Remember, a little goes a long way for both CBD balms and salves. To use, apply the product to the target area of your choice and rub in well. If you have inflamed knees and joints, don't be afraid to use on multiple parts of your body if needed. These products should not be applied directly to open wounds or opened blisters—just apply to your clean, dry skin. Turn to page 96 for a CBD Eucalyptus Mint Relief Balm recipe.

CBD Softgels & Supplements

If you're an athlete that pushes yourself daily (i.e., ultra-marathon runners) experimenting with higher doses of CBD (around 50 milligrams or more) might help you find relief. CBD softgels are a way to get higher doses, with the best products made from 100 percent all-natural CBD oil to best help with fitness training. To use, try taking the CBD softgel at night before bedtime as directed, and then proceed with your workout the following day. CBD supplements are also an option for casual athletes. The supplements tend to be a lower dose (between 15 to 30 milligrams of CBD), and they are most often combined with other healing ingredients such as ashwagandha root extract and L-theanine. Use as a daily supplement, beginning with one capsule a day (or your preference), and proceed with your normal workout routine.

CBD Powdered Mixes

If you love making protein shakes after a workout, CBD powdered mixes might be your new favorite ingredient. Think of these powder mixes the same way you'd think of normal protein powder. Add a packet to water, milk, or a smoothie after you exercise to see how it affects your recovery.

CBD & SEX

Getting intimate is another way to improve your self-care. If you've ever had a great orgasm, then you know just how it can help your worries fade away. Sex makes us feel good, which is due in part to the release of dopamine, which functions as a neurotransmitter that triggers the reward center in our brains. Spending intimate moments with your partner can also increase serotonin levels, the neurotransmitter that triggers happy feelings. When serotonin levels go up, dopamine levels go up, which makes sex an extremely pleasurable activity. There are many ways to incorporate CBD into the experience, to make these moments even better.

CBD is a tool that can be used before, during, or after sex, particularly for women; however, it may not provide the same euphoric and arousing side effects that you might find with THC intimacy products. Instead, CBD is great for inflammation, it reduces muscle tightness or spasms, and CBD oils can help keep things moist and slippery for maximum pleasure. Remember, not everyone will react the same way when using CBD. While some might feel a big difference, others might not experience any changes at all. It's up to you to determine what works best.

PRE-SEX

Before engaging in intercourse or self-pleasure, CBD can help you get in the mood by loosening up your body and releasing tension. For women, this means it might help relax the vulva and pelvic floor while providing moisture if you're using a CBD lubricant or CBD vaginal oil. It can also do wonders for menopausal discomfort. For men, using a CBD lubricant might help increase blood flow and nerve sensations, elevating sexual pleasure. Depending on what application you decide to use, there are benefits to using topicals, tinctures, smokables, or a combination.

DURING SEX

CBD lubricant or CBD vaginal oil can be easily re-applied during sex as you change positions with your partner. Just be sure to have the bottle nearby, so you're not interrupted.

POST-SEX

Above all, CBD is extremely beneficial for post-sex. For women, CBD vaginal oils can help with swelling and inflammation, which is a common side effect following intercourse. Have you ever felt sleepy after sex? Whether you're male or female, CBD can also help promote a good night's rest, which, in the end, ultimately benefits your sexual health and happiness.

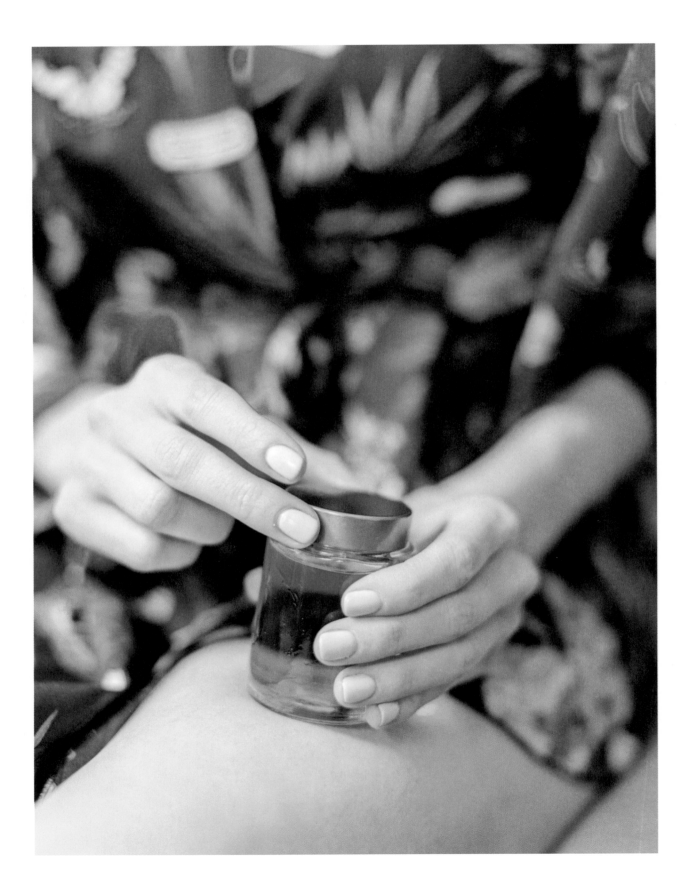

CBD INTIMACY PRODUCTS & HOW TO USE THEM

CBD lubricants aren't the only products that can spice things up in the bedroom. Breast oil, massage oil, and suppositories can also help in enhancing sexual pleasure. Below is an overview of each product and how to use them.

CBD Breast Oils & Serums

CBD breast oils and serums can be used during play and for self-care. The best brands blend cannabidiol with other therapeutic oils that soften, purify, and soothe the skin. If you have sore breasts, these products can help ease discomfort. To use, add a few drops of CBD breast oil or serum to the palms of your hand and begin to massage it in slowly. For men, you can also apply these oils to your chest and underarms to alleviate irritated skin.

CBD Massage Oil

While CBD lubricants can act as a massage oil when you're in the moment, actual CBD massage oil is a tool to integrate into your self-care and pleasure routine. Similar to the other topical products, CBD massage oil is helpful for joint pain, sore muscles, aches, and pains, and it can help with inflammation. To use, add an ample amount of oil to the palms of your hands. Rub together to create a warming sensation and then perform the massage. See page 98 for a Ylang-Ylang Spice Intimate CBD Massage Oil recipe.

CBD Suppositories

Quick and effective, CBD suppositories are an option for enhancing pleasure. Because suppositories avoid the digestive tract and absorb directly into the bloodstream via capillaries in the anal or vaginal passages, this application is a powerful way to integrate CBD into self-care and sex as it provides pathways to explore different sexual experiences. CBD suppositories can also be an effective treatment for lower back pain, menstrual cramps, and can help relieve many other ailments. Don't be shy! To use, insert the bolus 30 minutes before having sex, or simply insert, sit back, relax, and enjoy the enhanced medicinal properties.

GETTING INTIMATE WITH CBD

featuring Cyo Nystrom & Rachel Washtien, founders of Quim

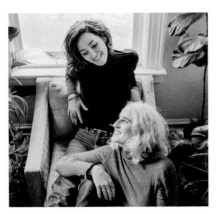

Cyo Nystrom and Rachel Washtien are experts when it comes to vaginal care. Quim is a self-care line for humans with vaginas and humans without vaginas who love vaginas. Cyo and Rachel make intimate products and pride themselves on their commitment to using plant-based ingredients to provide relief and pleasure to those who need it most. To learn more about their signature intimacy products, follow @its.quim or visit www.itsquim.com.

Cyo Nystrom & Rachel Washtien: "Our mission at Quim is to create products that deepen the connection that you have with your own body and empower you to care for it in the way that makes sense for you. Both CBD and THC can be worthwhile additions to your sex life. In our experience, CBD is particularly helpful in alleviating pain with penetration and promoting pelvic relaxation. It has been shown to be very helpful for people experiencing PTSD from sexual trauma.

CBD is generally more restorative and regenerative compared to the stimulating effects of THC. Post-sex maintenance is such an important part of one's sexual routine, and we absolutely think CBD products can improve your sex life. Less pain and more relaxation during and after sex? Who wouldn't want that?

What we've also learned through creating our vaginal health products is that hemp and cannabis affect everyone very differently, so while we can talk to what expected effects our products might have, it's really hard to say for sure. From personal experience and testimonials, we know that CBD can have a restorative effect, especially on people with vaginas. We like to remind people that you are the #1 expert on living in your own body. While we know what works for us, do what works best for you.

If you're thinking about making your own CBD intimacy products at home, we'd encourage you to think about your favorite ingredients and what you hope to get from that product. The next step would be to experiment. It might take a while to settle on something that works well for you, but make sure to keep track of the ingredients that you are working with and the heat levels that you're using to infuse the product. We recommend checking out the LEVO oil infuser for creating homemade plant-based products. Flip to page 50 in this book to learn more about this easy-to-use infusion machine. Enjoy!"

TIPS & TRICKS FOR CREATING SELF-CARE PRODUCTS AT HOME

Now that you're excited about CBD and self-care, it's time to make some healing products at home. The following tips and tricks will ensure that you create spa-quality facial masks, lip balm, bath soaks, and more—all incorporating your new favorite ingredient, CBD.

RECOMMENDED INGREDIENTS

In addition to cannabidiol, there are a few staple ingredients that you'll want to include in your recipes including terpene-inspired ingredients. For example, if you're looking to feel relaxed, using a product that's been infused with lavender or chamomile can induce sleepy sensations. If you're looking for relief after a big workout, rosemary or eucalyptus essential oils naturally provide restorative benefits. Calendula also acts as a powerful anti-inflammatory and is a fantastic ingredient to use in facial products or intimate oils.

You'll also want to stock up on different carrier oils and essential oils, plus some other ingredients such as Epsom salt and beeswax. Claudia Mata, founder of Vertly prefers to use fractionated MCT oil as a carrier for CBD because it's lightweight and absorbs quickly into the skin. She also likes pairing CBD with botanicals that complement its effectiveness such as arnica, calendula, comfrey root, yarrow, marjoram, and rosemary to help with body aches.

DOSING

When making CBD-infused remedy products, for the most part, you'll be creating topical products. Determining an exact dose with topicals can be challenging (especially if you're incorporating your own CBD infusions), but being precise is not as crucial as with edibles or drinkables. Be mindful of how much CBD you use because CBD products can be expensive. Look for affordable, clean options where you can use a greater amount without having to use all of your top-shelf products, or better yet, just infuse your own!

When making THC-infused products, remember that most topicals will not deliver intoxicating effects because they do not reach the bloodstream. Compared to food and drink, you can be more liberal when dosing THC in topicals, but be aware that if you are someone who may be drug tested, avoid THC topicals just to play it safe.

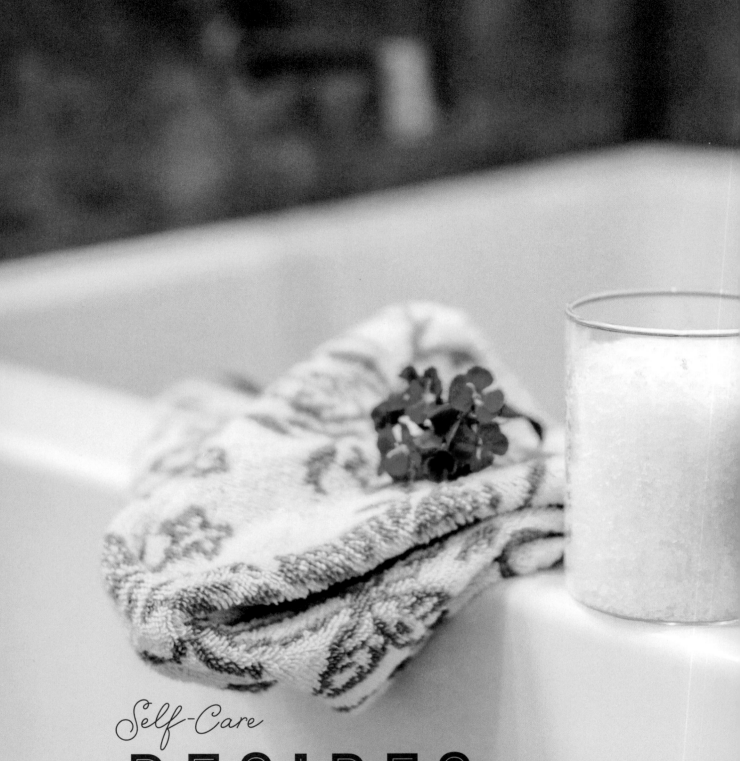

Self-Care

RECIPES

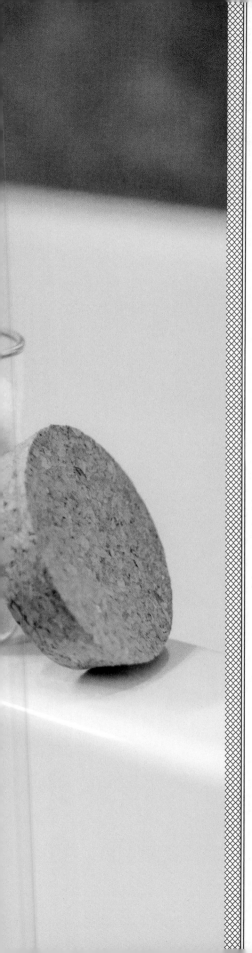

When it comes to CBD and self-care products, it's all about the oils! Not just CBD oil, but essential oils that are packed with healing benefits that soothe and take care of your body from head to toe. Believe it or not, honey is also a beneficial beauty product, particularly for the skin. With this in mind, the following recipes have been developed using a blend of CBD oils, essential oils, and CBD honey, plus other all-natural ingredients.

For best results, try infusing your base ingredients (CBD coconut oil, CBD fractionated coconut oil, and CBD honey) with CBD-rich flower so your body receives a broad range of cannabinoids, terpenes, and other healing compounds. If you don't have time to make these infusions, you can simply add professionally made CBD oil.

For the purposes of this book, the target doses that are indicated for DIY CBD ingredients are based on using Harle-Tsu flower that measured at a total of 15 percent CBD and 1 percent THC before decarboxylation. Refer back to page 52 for an overview on calculating dosages for the base ingredients that you'll be working with.

If you're using premade CBD products, the target dose is based on using a 30 milliliter bottle containing a total of 1,000 milligrams of CBD (or about 33 milligrams per dropper). Keep this in mind as you craft these recipes, but feel free to use whatever dosage best suits your needs.

When using essential oils for skin care, you should also be aware of a few safety tips. Always be sure to dilute an essential oil into a carrier oil before topical application. Typically a 2 percent dilution is recommended for use. Every self-care recipe in this book contains carrier oil (i.e., coconut, jojoba, argan, etc.), but note that everyone has different skin. If irritation occurs, discontinue use immediately.

Clear your calendar and prepare yourself for a fantastic at-home spa day. It's time for some rest and relaxation—you deserve it!

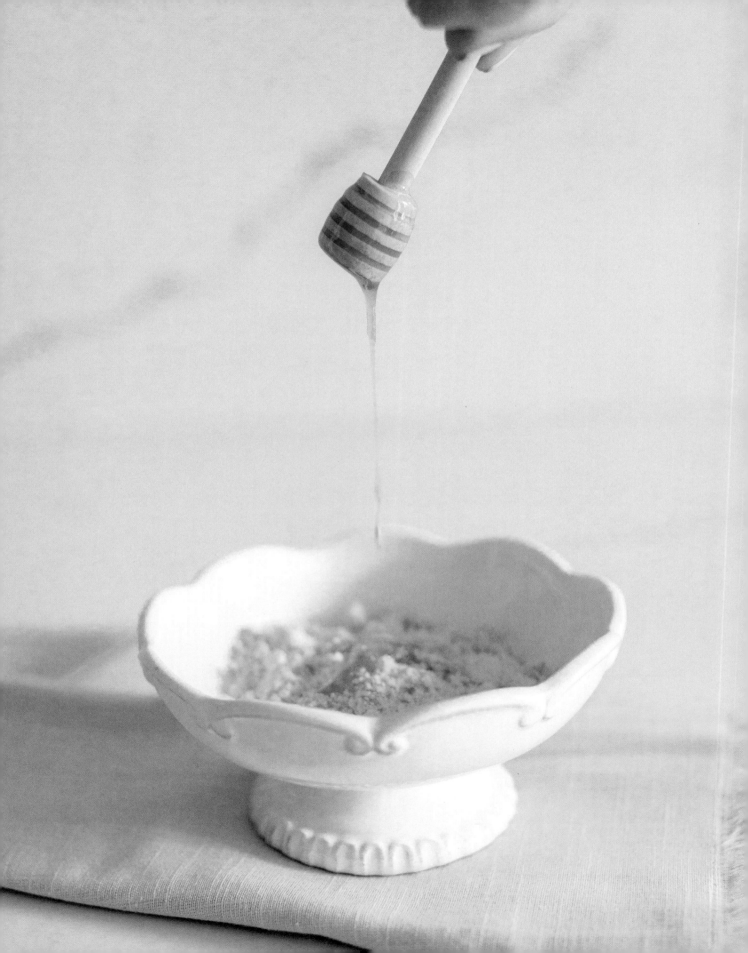

HONEY & OAT CBD FACIAL MASK

I love using honey for facial masks, particularly mixed with CBD. It provides antioxidants to combat the signs of aging, and it acts as a complexion enhancer that makes the skin glow. Oat powder is also a fantastic ingredient to use in facial masks because it contains saponins, which are natural cleansers that help control excess oil in the skin and remove pesky dirt that clogs pores. With the addition of soothing chamomile and rose oils, plus uplifting lemon oil, this mask will leave your skin radiant!

YIELD: 1 Mask	**TARGET DOSE:** 4 mg CBD | 0.3 mg THC per mask (using DIY CBD Coconut Oil Honey) or 16 mg CBD (using CBD Hemp Oil Honey, page 124)

EQUIPMENT
Spice grinder
Measuring spoons
Small bowl
Spoon

1 tablespoon (5 g) oats
1 tablespoon (14 g) CBD Coconut Oil Honey (page 124) or CBD Hemp Oil Honey (page 124)
¼ teaspoon jojoba oil
4 drops chamomile essential oil
1 drop rose essential oil
1 drop lemon essential oil

Using a spice grinder, grind the oats into a fine powder. The key here is making sure there are no clumps!

In a small bowl, combine the oat powder and honey—stir until it becomes a thick paste. Add the jojoba oil and the chamomile, rose, and lemon essential oils. Mix well.

To use: Cleanse your skin with warm water and dry with a towel. Pat on the facial mask, and apply in circular motions to exfoliate and massage into the skin. Allow the mask to dry for 10 minutes, then wash off with warm water and cleanser. Afterward, continue with your usual skin care routine. Your skin should feel extra soft and nourished with a special glow!

CBD COCONUT CHAMOMILE
LIP BALM

No matter what season it is, chapped, cracked lips are bound to happen. One of the best ways to prevent—and heal—this common ailment is to make sure you have a good lip balm to soothe your delicate lips. By combining CBD and a low dose of THC with jojoba oil and chamomile oil, you can naturally repair your precious pout. Jojoba oil is especially powerful for lip care because it's rich in fatty acids, which provides a wealth of hydration to the skin. Do your lips a favor and whip up a batch of this CBD lip balm.

YIELD: about 1 ounce (28 g)	**TARGET DOSE:** 28 mg CBD | 2 mg THC per batch (using CBD Coconut Oil, page 63) or 33 mg CBD (using commercially made CBD oil)

EQUIPMENT

One 8-ounce (240-ml) sterilized
    Mason jar
Measuring spoons
Small saucepan
Oven mitt
Small tin or glass container

1 tablespoon (10 g) beeswax pellets

**1 tablespoon (14 g) CBD Coconut Oil
(page 63)***

1 teaspoon jojoba oil

4 drops chamomile essential oil

1 drop calendula seed oil

1 drop lemongrass essential oil

In the Mason jar, combine the beeswax and CBD coconut oil. Fill a small saucepan about halfway with water. Place the *unsealed* Mason jar inside and begin to heat. Gently stir the mixture until both the beeswax and CBD coconut oil have fully melted.

Remove the Mason jar from the heat using an oven mitt. Add the jojoba, chamomile, calendula and lemongrass oils. Stir vigorously and then quickly pour the balm into a tin for storage. Once the CBD lip balm has firmed, use your fingernail to apply a thin layer to your chapped lips and enjoy.

NOTE

To infuse this recipe with commercially made CBD oil, use regular coconut oil when heating. Add 1 dropperful of the unflavored CBD oil of your choice (preferably made with fractionated coconut or MCT oil) when the essential oils are called for. Then follow the rest of the directions as written.

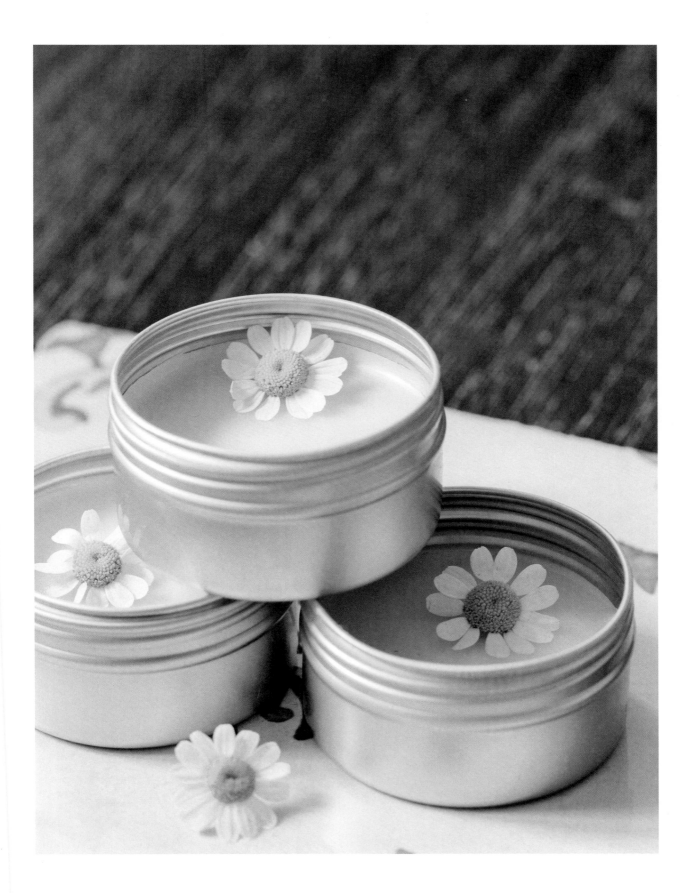

SMOKING VERSUS EATING/DRINKING THC AND CBD

If you've consumed infused edible or drinkable products before, you've most likely experienced some unique sensations that differ from smoking or vaping. For starters, if you ate an edible with THC in it, you might have felt stronger and more long-lasting side effects than hitting a joint. Conversely, if you've vaped, smoked, or dabbed CBD, you might feel stronger effects than if you were to eat/drink CBD-infused foods or beverages. There is a reason for this. Smoking versus eating/drinking THC and CBD impacts you differently. Let's break it down.

First, let's focus on THC (a.k.a. delta-9-tetrahydrocannabinol) because the effects are more obvious and we have a longer history to examine. Depending on what consumption method you choose, your body absorbs THC differently because of the way it converts it into 11-Hydroxy-Δ9-tetrahydrocannabinol (11-Hydroxy-THC) in your liver. If you are new to 11-Hydroxy-THC, it is metabolic derivative of THC and an entirely different compound that's formed by the human body once THC is processed. Unlike THC, this compound does not naturally exist in the cannabis plant. When 11-Hydroxy-THC is formed, potency levels can vary greatly depending on whether you consume cannabis as an edible (converts at high levels) or smoke it (converts at low levels). While some people might have a high THC tolerance while smoking, this does not mean they'll have a high tolerance for edibles.

When smoked or vaporized, THC passes through the lungs before entering the bloodstream, where little metabolism takes place. The THC that remains in your blood is available to go to the liver, where it is converted to 11-Hydroxy-THC and other metabolites, but at extremely low levels. Because such a small amount of THC converts, you'll most likely not feel any effects from the 11-Hydroxy-THC after smoking. Instead, Δ-9-THC kicks in as fast as 30 to 90 seconds. Depending on the person and how much was inhaled, the high can last between 1 to 2 hours. Generally, the effects of smoked or vaporized cannabis come quicker and diminish faster than eating or drinking THC-infused products.

When ingested orally, THC passes through the stomach and metabolizes in the liver, which converts it to 11-hydroxy-THC. Depending on how many milligrams you ate, 11-Hydroxy-THC has the potential for creating a more intense high. Digestion isn't the fastest process, so effects might be felt within 20 to 45 minutes after drinking an infused beverage or between 1 to 2 hours after eating infused cuisine. Knowing your metabolism and being patient are key for any edible experience. Once side effects kick in, the high can last for up to 8 hours depending on how much is consumed. Be sure to be mindful about your surroundings, and never drive after consuming an edible or drinkable.

(continued)

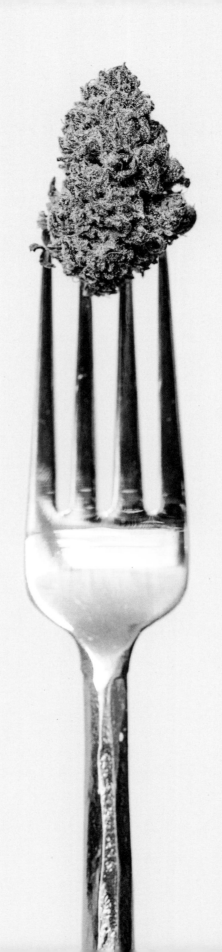

So, what about CBD? Are there differences between smoking it and eating/drinking it?

As we discussed on page 24, the bioavailability of CBD depends on the consumption method and concentration of the cannabidiol that you are consuming. When smoked or vaped, CBD is inhaled through the lungs, quickly entering the bloodstream and delivering a high bioavailability rate, providing your body with higher amounts of CBD. So far, studies have shown that smoking, vaping, or dabbing might be a more effective solution for taking CBD rather than oral consumption methods (i.e., CBD edibles, CBD beverages).

When ingested orally, CBD must pass through the gut and liver, which filters out portions of CBD during the metabolic and digestive process. CBD's bioavailability is reduced because the liver decreases the concentration of bioactive compounds before they have a chance to enter the bloodstream. Essentially, not all of the CBD you consume via food or drink will affect your body.

For those looking to use CBD for medical purposes, using sublinguals or concentrates might be a better option if you are seeking higher bioavailability rates. Keep this in mind when you are infusing CBD into your food and beverages. Lower dosages might not be as effective, because your body will only absorb a small portion of what you consumed.

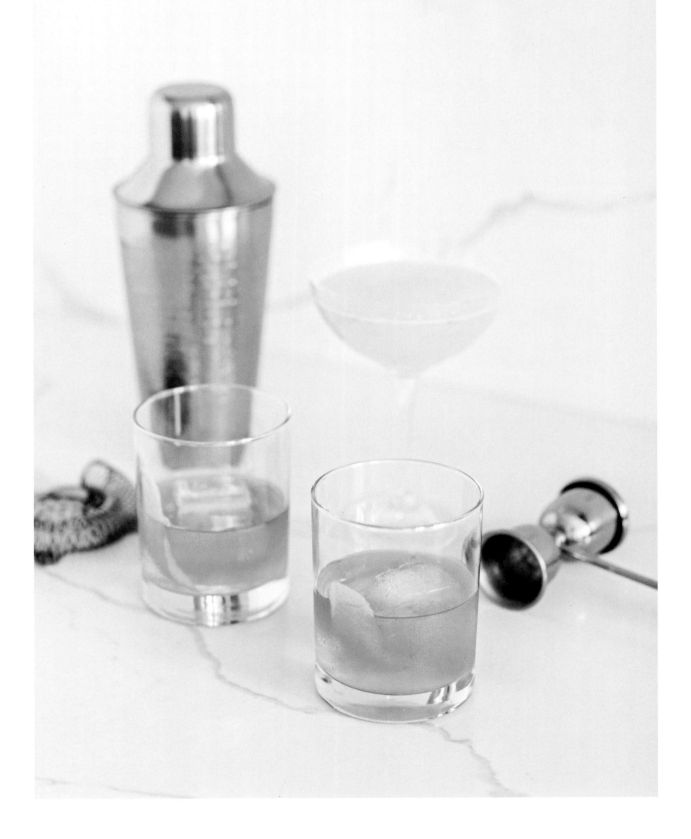

COMBINING CBD & ALCOHOL

For anyone who's tried mixing THC and alcohol, you know there's a fine balance between feeling great to feeling dizzy and sick. When mixing, you should always follow the golden rule, "start low, go slow." Safe and responsible cannabis consumption should always be top of mind, especially when another intoxicant is introduced into your body.

While CBD does not have the same intoxicating effects as THC, the interactions between cannabidiol and alcohol have not been thoroughly researched. Some studies are showing that consuming both together doesn't seem to have any immediate adverse side effects. Still, knowing that there is not much concrete research to rely on, it is best to play it safe and not go overboard. Pay close attention to how your body reacts after consuming. Avoid mixing CBD with other medications. And above all, do not drive or operate machinery after consuming CBD cocktails.

These same rules apply to THC, but be even more cautious and aware of how you're feeling. THC is a powerful plant medicine. If used correctly and responsibly, it can be an enjoyable experience. If used incorrectly, the combination of THC and alcohol can greatly impair you. John Korkidis, founder of the popular cannabis mixology blog *Chron Vivant* and Proposition Cocktail Co., tries to avoid combining known intoxicating cannabinoids, like THC, with alcohol altogether. Instead, most of his recipes leverage a broad-spectrum of cannabinoids that are rich in CBD but have very little, to no, THC. If you do decide to combine the two, do not drive. Always take precautions, and don't overdo it.

Warren Bobrow, expert mixologist and author of the hit book, *Cannabis Cocktails, Mocktails & Tonics* suggests to start slow if you are planning to mix with THC. Experiment with low doses to find the right balance, and don't mix with high-proof alcohol for a cocktail.

If CBD cocktails aren't right for you, don't fret. There are many other ways you can enjoy the benefits of CBD minus the alcohol. In the coming pages, you'll learn how to create the perfect mocktail along with CBD-infused coffee, iced tea, and much more.

MIXING CBD INTO YOUR FAVORITE DRINKS

There are many, many ways to mix CBD into beverages, but there are a few methods that are widely accepted as working better than others. The three most common techniques include making an infusion, using a CBD oil or alcohol-based tincture, or combining isolate powder with beverage recipes. Regardless of the technique you decide to use, all of these approaches can be done successfully at home.

INFUSIONS

As you learned on page 51, an infusion is a process of extracting chemical compounds (THC and CBD) from cannabis or hemp material in a solvent such as alcohol, oil, butter, or other fat-based liquids, by allowing the material to be suspended in the solvent over time. There are many methods you can use including sous vide, stovetop, slow cooker, or an infusion device. Because CBD and THC bind with fats and alcohol (not water), you'll want to use one of these substances as the foundation of your extraction. Let's run through a few simple infusions you should be familiar with as we continue with this chapter.

Alcohol Infusions

When making CBD cocktails or mocktails, creating an infusion is a great way to incorporate cannabidiol into your recipes. Grain alcohol (a.k.a. ethanol) is the source of extraction for this method and can either be heated or used at room temperature to extract terpenes and cannabinoids from CBD-rich cannabis flower.

Heating increases the efficiency of the extraction, but it is also more dangerous as alcohol is flammable and has a low boiling point. If you decide to use a heating method, never use a gas stove and do not seal the Mason jar. Also, whatever you do, keep temperatures below 170°F (77°C)—alcohol flames at this point.

To make a heated infusion, use a hot plate (no flame) to heat the alcohol and cannabis flower in an unsealed sterilized Mason jar on low for about 45 minutes. Set up your cooking station near a window to allow clean air into the room as the alcohol burns off.

For room-temperature infusions, simply combine the alcohol and dried cannabis flower in a sterilized Mason jar and store in a dark pantry or cabinet for up to 30 days. Occasionally agitate the mixture to help with the extraction process.

Whatever method you choose, you'll want to use cheesecloth and a fine-mesh strainer to remove solids from the infused alcohol before serving. The majority of your favorite liquors will work for this type of infusion, but if you're looking to extract unique flavors and if you want the infused alcohol to be drinkable (compared to an Everclear alcohol-based tincture) vodka, gin, light rum, and tequila are good alcohols to use. You can also infuse darker spirits, but because the flavors are already so rich, you may not be able to perceive the terpene

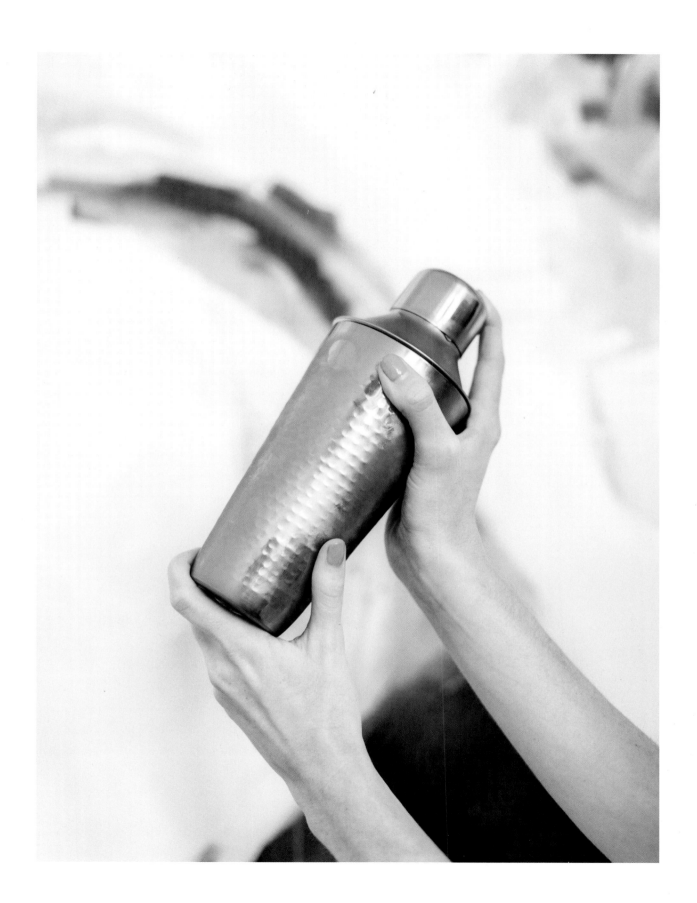

profiles or flavors of the infusion. Not everyone enjoys the taste of cannabis, so this might not be an issue for you. For an alcohol-based infusion recipe, see page 113.

Honey & Simple Syrups

Mixing infused honey and simple syrups into beverages is a great way to add CBD into your favorite drinks. As substitutes for processed sugar and artificial sweeteners, both of these substances are a must-have for CBD beverages and are easy to infuse.

With honey, you can make an infusion by adding CBD coconut oil, hemp oil, or isolate powder. When adding a CBD oil, use a blender to vigorously mix the oil into the honey, creating a fast and effective infused product. Be aware that separation will occur over time, but because honey is so viscous, it is more resistant to this change. CBD isolate powders are less susceptible to separation if infused correctly, which involves melting the powder into a small amount of MCT oil (or oil of your choice) at 140°F to 150°F (60°C to 66°C) and mixing it into the honey over low heat to set the emulsion.

Once you create an infused honey, you can add it smoothies, hot tea, on top of yogurt, and so much more. After consumption, honey enters directly into the bloodstream, providing almost instantaneous effects. For those of you that follow Ayurvedic traditions, you already know that honey is one of the foundations of administering herbal medicine. For a CBD honey recipe, see page 124.

If you are planning to make CBD mocktails or cocktails, you'll also want to have a CBD simple syrup on hand. I am a big fan of using agave nectar as a base for simple syrup recipes because it is a plant-based food that is a natural alternative to processed sugar. It also dissolves easily in cold drinks, making it a perfect choice to add to iced tea and lemonade. For a CBD simple syrup recipe, see page 126.

Fat-Based Liquids

Because CBD and THC are fat soluble, these cannabinoids and other medicated molecules bind with fat-based liquids easily. Creating infused milk using cream, high-fat dairy milk, coconut milk, or soymilk is an easy way to combine cannabinoids into drinks, particularly coffee and tea. You can create an infusion by adding a CBD isolate powder to the milk of your choice and mixing over low heat, or by infusing decarboxylated CBD-rich cannabis flower into the fat-based liquid by directly combining the two in a small saucepan and heat on low (around 160°F [71°C]) for 1 hour. I do not recommend adding CBD oil to these infusions because of the risk of separation and uneven distribution. For a fat-based recipe, see Cinnamon-Spiced Milk recipe on page 129.

Fat-Washing

Fat-washing is a method of infusion that relies on the extraction that occurs between fat flavor molecules and alcohol. Ethanol solutions are best for this method because they have the ability to extract and dissolve fatty flavors. When combined, fatty oils and alcohol separate; however, your extraction process has begun. The alcohol begins to break down the fat, leaving behind delicious, fat-flavored alcohol (think bacon-flavored vodka). Fat-washing is a successful technique when it comes to extracting cannabinoids because, as you've learned, THC and CBD love binding with fat-based and alcohol-based solutions. This process allows these compounds to be extracted and infused into the spirit you are working with, creating a base for infused beverages.

To create a simple fat-washed infusion at home, simply combine 4 to 8 ounces (120 to 240 ml) of CBD or THC-infused olive oil or coconut oil with 750 milliliters of the alcohol of your choice in a large sterilized Mason jar (I enjoy CBD-infused coconut oil mixed with rum). Shake vigorously for a couple of minutes, and then set the mixture in the freezer to chill overnight. The next morning, remove the liquid by poking a hole in the hardened fat that has risen to the top and strain before serving.

ISOLATE POWDER

If you decide to use isolate powder in beverages, it is a fast and potent way to integrate CBD into your regimen; however, be aware that you are missing out on the terpenes and the other cannabinoids that enhance CBD's therapeutic properties. Isolates do allow you to administer higher doses of CBD, unlike some premade hemp CBD oils and tinctures that cap out around 5 to 10 milligrams per serving. Nonetheless, when compared to full-spectrum products, isolates require very high doses to be effective.

CBD isolate powder is not water soluble. If added to a beverage without infusing properly, the isolate will float on the top of your drink. Because isolates are odorless and flavorless, you can integrate them into the beverage of your choice by melting them into a liquid between 140°F to 150°F (60°C to 66°C). However, if you are creating smoothies or other blended drinks, heating doesn't matter as much. Just be sure to use a scale to measure your desired dose before putting the isolate into the blender.

TINCTURES

One of the most common—and quick—ways to add CBD to beverages is by adding a few drops of a professionally made or homemade CBD tincture into your recipe. If you're using an alcohol-based tincture, it will blend seamlessly into drinks. On the other hand, mixologists across the nation have mixed reviews on using CBD oil drops. Some prefer to add oil-based tinctures because the CBD oil that floats on top of the liquid can add a pleasant complexity to certain drinks, act as a decorative garnish, and contribute to a pleasurably thick mouthfeel. Other professionals believe that oil-based CBD drops can overpower the flavor of the drink and are not a reliable way to receive the benefits of CBD—a good deal of the oil can end up at the bottom of your glass. It's really up to you to decide what method you'd like to use; however, most pros will recommend alcohol-based tinctures and or CBD Bitters (page 113).

CREATING CBD BITTERS AT HOME

featuring John Korkidis, founder of *Chron Vivant* & Proposition Cocktail Co.

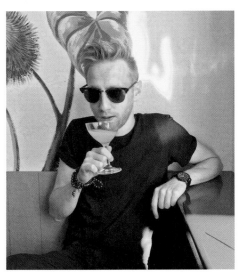

John Korkidis is a San Francisco–based cannabis mixologist, educator, and founder of Chron Vivant. *His online platform explores refined cannabis and hemp cocktails, bitters, and other potent potable recipes for the modern Bon Vivant, hence the name! John is also the founder of Proposition Cocktail Co., an all-natural nonalcoholic cocktails and adaptogenic mood-enhancers line that adds an elevated twist to a variety of beverages. Follow John @chronvivant and @proposition.co or visit ChronVivant.com.*

John Korkidis: "Once found in early apothecaries, cannabis bitters and tinctures were widely reputed for their medicinal effects, up until the early 1900s when America's attitude toward cannabis began to change. Bitters differ from tinctures in that bitters are typically used to add layers of nuanced flavor and pungent aromatics to drinks, whereas tinctures usually add just a singular flavor profile. Cannabis- and hemp-derived CBD bitters, like other bitters, are meant to be more of an aromatic flavoring agent than an intoxicant; which is great for those looking to microdose.

Making your own DIY CBD bitters is as easy as infusing your choice of botanicals, roots, barks, fruits, and herbs (and yes even "herb") in a high-proof spirit or grain alcohol.

Applied in dashes, this bitters recipe is inspired by the classic flavor profile of Angostura, used to craft cocktails such as the Manhattan and the old-fashioned. You can easily adjust this base recipe with other ingredients to create a myriad of bitters flavors, such as orange, lavender, celery, etc. Don't stress if you don't have all the ingredients on hand; almost everything listed is readily available online. Just like cooking, you can also substitute many of the botanicals, roots, and herbs listed for things that are local to your region. Have fun experimenting."

CHRON VIVANT CBD BITTERS

YIELD: about 16 ounces (475 ml)

EQUIPMENT
Two 32-ounce (940-ml) sterilized
    Mason jars
Cheesecloth
Fine-mesh strainer
Saucepan

7–10 grams organic CBD-rich cannabis

1 fresh orange peel, cut into thin strips

2 whole dried orange leaves (organic
    if possible)

4 cardamom pods, cracked

1½ cinnamon sticks

1 whole star anise

1 whole vanilla bean, halved and
    shaved

2 tablespoons (12 g) dried orange peel,
    chopped

¼ cup (40 g) dried sour cherries

¾ teaspoon cloves

¾ teaspoon cassia chips

¾ teaspoon dried gentian root

¾ teaspoon dried angelica root

2½ cups (600 ml) high-proof bourbon
    or rye (preferably rye), plus more
    as needed

1 cup (240 ml) filtered drinking water

2 ounces (60 ml) rich simple syrup

Step 1 (crucial step): Decarboxylate your cannabis (page 48) to activate the CBDA and THCA into CBD and THC. Be careful not to excessively heat as you can easily damage and degrade the CBD and THC.

Step 2: Place your dry ingredients in a Mason jar. Pour in 2½ cups (600 ml) of bourbon, or enough so that your ingredients are covered. Seal the jar and store it at room temperature, away from direct sunlight, for 12 to 16 days. Gently agitate the jar every 1 to 2 days. After about 2 weeks, you should be able to taste the aromatics, botanicals, and herbs maturing together. When you feel your infusion is ready, it's time to finish the product.

Step 3: Strain the liquid through cheesecloth lining a fine-mesh strainer into a clean jar; be sure to save the leftover solids. Repeat this until all the remaining sediment is removed.

Transfer the solids to a small clean saucepan, barely cover with the water, and bring to a boil.

Once boiling, cover the saucepan, reduce the heat to low and simmer for 8 to 10 minutes. Remove from the heat and let cool completely. When cool, add the liquids and solids to a clean jar and store for 5 to 7 days. Agitate the bottle every few days.

Step 4: Strain the liquid as before to remove all the solids and sediment. At this point, you can discard both the solids and sediment. Add this newly stained liquid to the original bitters base solution. And add the rich simple syrup.

Technically you are ready to go, but I suggest you let the infusion rest for 2 to 3 days before decanting into smaller jars and using, storing, or giving away as gifts.

(continued)

Don't worry if there is some minor sediment or residue, although you could continue to strain if desired. Otherwise, that's it! Your hard work and patience has paid off. Your new batch of bitters should last a lifetime, but for optimal flavor and aromatics, I recommend you use within a year.

Potency for every 2 to 3 dashes of bitters is approximately 5 to 15 milligrams of CBD, depending on the cannabis strain and the amount that you used.

Keep in mind that this basic recipe lends itself to improvisation. Just like cooking, mix and match your favorite flavors and have fun making it your own. The more you continue to experiment, the more comfortable you'll become and the better your bitters will taste!

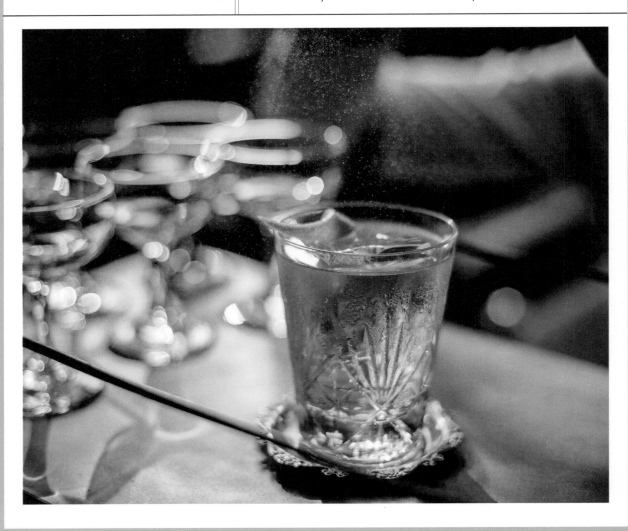

TIPS & TRICKS FOR CREATING INFUSED BEVERAGES

Whether you are making a simple infusion or blending up a more complex CBD cocktail, the following tools and best practices will help you maneuver your way around a variety of drink recipes, including the recipes highlighted in this book. These helpful suggestions and ideas come from my collaboration with three of the most highly trained professionals in the industry, Rachel Burkons of Altered Plates, John Korkidis of *Chron Vivant*, and Warren Bobrow, The Cocktail Whisperer. We are thrilled to share our insider secrets with you.

CONSIDER FLAVORS

When making an infused beverage, finding fresh and flavorful ingredients is key. Because CBD products can often have green notes, incorporating terpene-inspired aromas and flavors will play well with both cannabis and hemp characteristics.

Rachel Burkons, an expert cannabis/CBD mixologist based in Los Angeles, recommends using terpene-inspired fruits, herbs, and spices in infused drink recipes. Rosemary, thyme, cinnamon, clove, lemon, lime, grapefruit, mango, pineapple, blueberries, and blackberries are a good starting point. She also recommends using gin. While there are many styles of gin, choosing a botanical-driven brand is best because hemp and cannabis aromas and flavors intertwine perfectly.

Cannabis mixologist, John Korkidis, recommends using infused garnishes and aromatic terpenes to make elevated beverages. By using these ingredients, you can incorporate cannabis and CBD into drinks without adulterating the classic base recipes.

DOSING STANDARDS

As discussed, research is showing that CBD is safe when consumed at higher doses; however, it is best to start on the low side of the dosage range and adjust upward over time until the desired effect is achieved. That is just as true with beverages as with other methods of consumption. Here are some other recommendations on how to find your ideal dose when mixing CBD (or THC) into beverages:

While there are no standards for dosing, generally, between 15 to 30 milligrams of CBD or between 1 to 5 milligrams of THC per beverage is a safe place to start for beginners. Remember, you will not get high with CBD!

If you are using a professionally made CBD tincture to infuse your beverage recipe, start with the brand's recommended dose per serving. Before mixing it into your drink, try a single serving of the CBD on its own. After consuming, see how you feel and then go up or down in milligrams depending on your needs. If you're using a product with THC, start with a low dose (2.5 milligrams max) and see how you feel. Adjust up or down accordingly.

With traditional cocktails and mocktails, it's common to have more than one drink. But when consuming infused beverages, drinking multiple is not recommended. Keep track of your milligram intake—especially if you are drinking THC-infused beverages. Do not overdo it!

MISTAKES TO AVOID

Don't worry, we've all made rookie mistakes when trying something new, and that also applies to learning how to consume CBD and THC safely and responsibly. Mixing CBD into drinks has its own challenges. To make life easier, here are some common mistakes to avoid:

Mistake #1: Purchasing the first product you see on the internet.

Take the time to educate yourself on what quality products are out there, and learn the differences and nuances between each brand. Some top resources for CBD information include Project CBD, *Leafly*, *Nice Paper*, among others. Also, understand what full spectrum means (page 22) and why this is important when sourcing your CBD. In addition, Warren Bobrow recommends that you pay close attention to how much you are paying for CBD. A big mistake would be to pay too much for something that's not effective. Avoid cheap online websites, and find a reliable brand that's not trying to overcharge you.

Mistake #2: Not integrating the CBD into your drink properly.

The majority of CBD products that you'll see on the market are CBD oils. Whether from hemp or cannabis, oil is not the easiest product to mix into drinks because it will separate if not integrated correctly. To ensure you are creating a well-made infused beverage (not simply adding drops of oil on top), remember these three simple integration strategies:

If you're using oil, emulsify cannabidiol into your beverage by muddling the CBD with different fruits, herbs, and a little simple syrup. Once you're done muddling, add the rest of your ingredients to the beverage, and voilà! You've successfully integrated the CBD into your beverage. Oil-based tinctures also work well for frothy beverages and coffee, but be careful how you use them. Sometimes, without the proper emulsification, the oil can rise to the surface of a drink affecting the mouthfeel and desired taste.

When making an elevated CBD or THC mixer for certain recipes that don't call for a fat- or ethanol-based solvent, you can use lecithin or vegetable glycerin during the infusion process to help absorb CBD or THC. Lecithin is a fat that can be found in many foods, including sunflowers, soybeans, and egg yolks (sunflower is the best type to use for your infusions). It is also used as a food and drink additive because it keeps certain ingredients from separating (in this case, it helps prevent CBD from separating). You can also use vegetable glycerin in your recipes, which is particularly useful if you're making an infused simple syrup (page 126). Glycerin accelerates the uptake of CBD or THC in your digestive system, facilitating a quicker onset. Whether you're using lecithin or vegetable glycerin, it's recommended to add 1 to 2 tablespoons (11 to 22 g, or 15 to 30 ml, respectively) of either depending on what your recipe calls for. Both of these products can be found online or head to your local health food store to find a reliable brand.

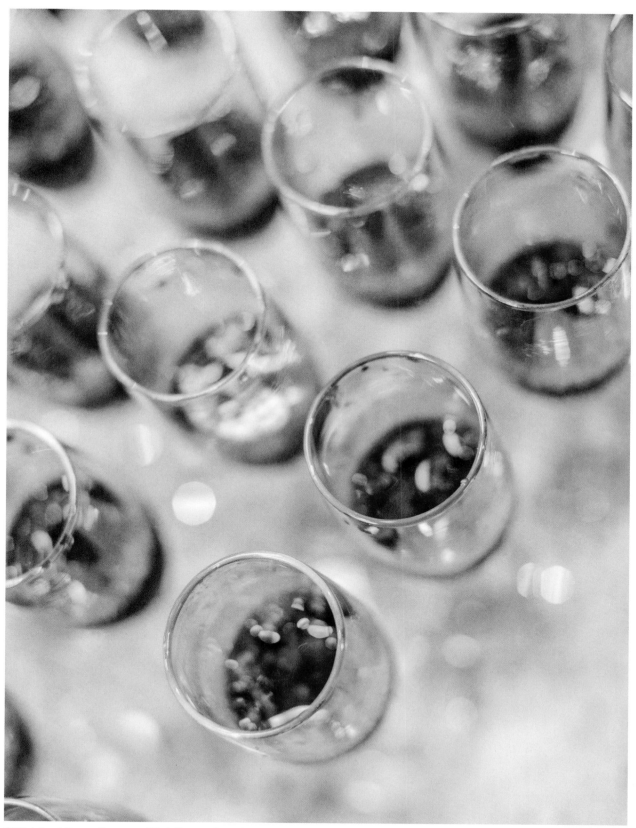

CBD-infused Orange Blossom and Early Summer Berry Spritzer served at The Herb Somm's Feast of the Flowers event.

You can always use a shaker tin to integrate CBD into your favorite drinks. The more you vigorously shake, the better the CBD will mix into the other liquids. If you use an oil, be prepared for separation to occur over time, but you can easily re-emulsify but giving it a good shake.

Mistake #3: Forgetting to label your infusions.

When creating infusions at home, it is crucial that you label everything that's been infused. Whether it's CBD or THC, be sure to put a piece of tape on the lid of your Mason jars and mark what the infusion is and how many milligrams it contains. If you live with other people, this step is even more vital. If you live with children, take extra precautions and be sure to store your infusions in a safe place where they cannot be accessed.

SERVING TIPS

The best thing you can do when serving infused beverages is to make sure everyone knows what is what. Be sure to label everything and communicate with your guests throughout the event or social gathering to remind them that the beverages are infused. Before guests arrive, check in with the group to see what their dosage preferences are. Not everyone will want to consume CBD, so be sure to have non-infused drink options available as well. If you are planning to serve multiple drinks infused with CBD, be sure to remember that the milligrams will add up. Keep track of the cumulative amount that will be served and communicate this with your guests. This is a crucial step that I always incorporate into my own events.

If you've prepared an elevated mixer, be sure it is easy to re-emulsify. As we've learned, CBD oil can separate from other liquids, so be sure to have the ability to easily mix it up again if necessary.

If you decide to add CBD tincture drops to mocktails or cocktails, you can set up a DIY bar and have your guests infuse their own drinks based on their preferred dosages. If you're just serving CBD, you don't need to worry about anyone overdoing it; however, be sure to provide signage that lists how many milligrams per milliliter of CBD are in your featured tincture blend.

Another fun idea is to have terpene-inspired garnishes available, such as juniper berries, mint, rosemary, or lavender, for your guests to put in their drinks. This is a great conversation starter and a fun way to integrate the topic of terpenes into your party or event. You'll be impressed with the creations your guests come up with.

Finally, when serving CBD drinks, consider presentation. Make sure they are attractive looking and don't be afraid to try new things. CBD beverages are a fantastic way to educate your friends and family, so have fun with it.

THE PERFECT CBD MOCKTAIL
Terpene Highballs

featuring Rachel Burkons of Altered Plates

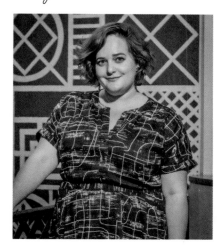

Rachel Burkons is the co-founder of Los Angeles–based hospitality company, Altered Plates. After spending more than a decade in the wine and spirits industry as the cannabis editor for national publication The Clever Root, *and the VP/associate publisher for sister publications* The Tasting Panel *and* The SOMM Journal, *Rachel is an expert mixologist and one of the leading voices in exploring the connection between food, drinks, and cannabis. With close ties to top chefs, mixologists, and sommelier tastemakers across the country, she is also a leading educator and hospitality consultant who specializes in the cannabis space. For more cannabis cocktail and hospitality tips, follow Rachel @smokesipsavor.*

Rachel Burkons: "When it comes to the flavors of cannabis, I say this: Lean in! Cannabis—and many high-quality CBD oils and tinctures—can offer a wealth of unique flavors, all derived from our favorite flavor and feeling molecules, terpenes! But terpenes are also the building blocks of flavor in many of the foods you probably either already have, or have easy access to, such as limes, black peppercorn, rosemary, and mango. Combining these two flavor bombs—terpene-rich CBD oils and fresh herbs and fruits—results in a series of easy at-home spritzers I call Terpene Highballs.

In the realm of cocktails, the Highball, classically comprised of whiskey and a soda mixer, is one of the simplest ways to showcase a quality spirit. Similarly, by reaching for sparkling water, these Terpene Highballs not only celebrate the flavors of cannabis or hemp in CBD tinctures, but also keep things health and wellness focused. If you're feeling a bit naughty (as I tend to), feel free to add an ounce or two of your favorite spirit to one of these recipes. I've included a suggested spirit pairing, but these spritzers are meant to be seasonal, casual, and flavorful, so get inspired by what you smell and taste at the farmer's market and let your palate guide you as you create your own Terpene Highball recipe."

BLACK PEPPER & BERRY
(beta-Caryophyllene) HIGHBALL

Turning to classic flavor combinations like sweet-and-spicy works wonders for intense, peppery beta-Caryophyllene. This terpene lingers at the back of the throat when smoking cannabis, and you'll find it hits the same spot on your palate when consumed via food or beverage. Double down on the pepper if you want an intense, spicy experience!

YIELD: **1** serving	**TARGET DOSE:** 15 mg CBD (using a commercially made CBD tincture)

EQUIPMENT
Shaker tin
Muddler
Collins glass

5 strawberries (plus more for garnish)

CBD tincture of your choice (15 mg CBD or your preferred dose)

1½ ounces (45 ml) fresh lemon juice

1 ounce (30 ml) Black Pepper Simple Syrup (see sidebar)

Ice, for serving

Soda water, for topping

1 ounce (15 ml) rhubarb tea liqueur (optional)

Cut the strawberries in half. In a shaker tin, muddle the strawberries, CBD tincture, lemon juice, and simple syrup. Pour over ice and top with soda water. Garnish with a strawberry slice.

To add alcohol, add the rhubarb tea liqueur to your shaker tin and proceed with the directions above.

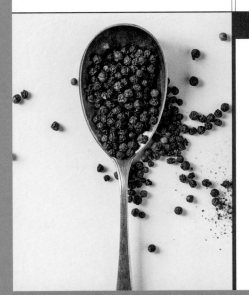

BLACK PEPPER SIMPLE SYRUP

To make black pepper simple syrup: Bring one part water to a boil; add one part sugar. Once the sugar is dissolved, add 1 tablespoon (8 g) whole black peppercorns. Leave the peppercorns to infuse, to taste. When cool, cover and refrigerate for up to 2 weeks. Strain before using.

MANGO MOJITO *(myrcene)* HIGHBALL

Terpene highballs are intended to be an easy way to incorporate CBD into your daily routine. Mango is a fantastic fruit to use because, like cannabis, it contains elevated levels of the terpene myrcene. Myrcene provides a broad spectrum of therapeutic benefits, which allows for maximum healing—the perfect addition to any CBD-infused drink!

YIELD: **4** servings	**TARGET DOSE:** 15 mg CBD per drink (using a commercially made CBD tincture)

EQUIPMENT
Blender
4 Collins glasses

---

2 large mangoes, cored, peeled, and diced

¼ cup (48 g) fresh mint leaves (plus more for garnish)

2 ounces (60 ml) fresh lime juice

1½ ounces (45 ml) Honey Simple Syrup (see sidebar)

2 cups (480 ml) purified cold water, plus more as needed

Ice, for serving

CBD tincture of your choice (60 mg CBD or your preferred dose)

Soda water, for topping

1½ ounces (45 ml) white rum (optional)

Lime wheels, for garnish

In a blender, combine the mango, mint, lime juice, simple syrup, and cold water. Add more water as needed until blended into a smooth purée. Cover and chill until cold.

Pour the mango purée over ice into the Collins glasses. Stir in one-quarter of the CBD tincture (15 mg per drink). Top with soda water. Add the rum (if using) and stir to incorporate. Garnish with a lime wheel and mint sprig.

A note about batching your drinks: Batching mocktails and cocktails is a great way to incorporate cannabis into your entertaining experiences—but the best way to ensure consistent, safe consumption of any cannabinoid is to dose each drink individually. Once you've whipped up a batch of this simple alcohol-free spritzer, teach your guests how to determine their perfect dosage and be mindful if they're consuming more than one!

HONEY SIMPLE SYRUP

Honey is a great flavor conductor for terpenes, and different honey varieties may be used to enhance the terpene mocktail experience. Orange blossom honey, for example, is known for a light citrus-kissed flavor that's a beautiful match with limonene. Buckwheat honey, known for its dark, funky flavors, is a wonderful carrier that stands up to the sometimes overwhelming "green" notes in some tinctures.

Experiment with honeys that work for you. Just follow this basic formula for any honey simple syrup recipe: Heat one part water until hot; add one part honey. Stir. Cool, cover, and refrigerate for up to 2 weeks.

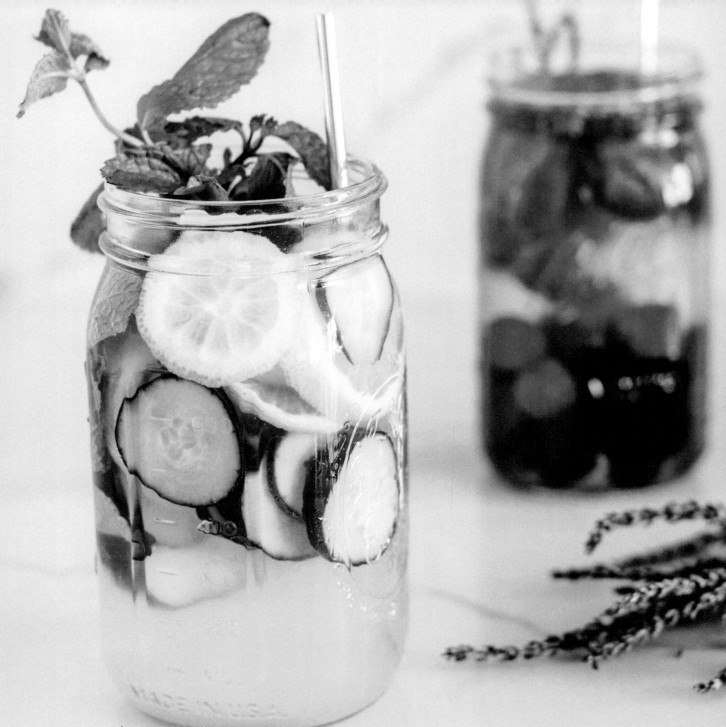

Beverage

RECIPES

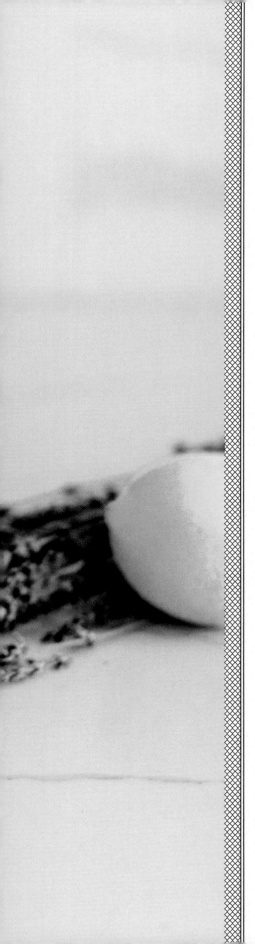

The following recipes have been developed using a variety of products. For the infusion recipes using CBD-rich cannabis, I used Harle-Tsu flower that measured at a total of 15 percent CBD and 1 percent THC before decarboxylation. These numbers will differ depending on the strain and source of the product that you use, so be sure to calculate your own CBD/THC milligrams per serving before making your infusion (see page 52 for at-home dosage calculations).

The target dose per serving listed in this chapter can be used as a baseline, but know that your final outcome will vary if you're using your own infusions. Do your best to make an accurate estimate, and always sample each batch with conservative tastings before serving to others.

If you're using commercially made CBD products, the target dose is based on using a 30 milliliter bottle containing a total of 1,000 milligrams of CBD (or about 33 milligrams CBD per dropper or about 17 milligrams CBD per ½ dropper). If you'd rather use a higher or lower dose of CBD than what's listed in this chapter, by all means, use the dosage that works best for your needs. Keep this in mind as you craft these drinkables.

I hope you enjoy this collection of my favorite CBD-Infused beverage recipes. Have fun, be safe, and enjoy responsibly!

CBD HONEY, TWO WAYS

There are many ways to infuse honey at home. What follows are two different techniques using DIY coconut oil made with CBD-rich flower (see page 63) and commercially made CBD hemp oil. You'll be using oil in both of these recipes, so be aware that separation can occur over time. If this is the case, re-emulsify your honey by blending before serving.

CBD COCONUT OIL HONEY

YIELD: 1 cup (340 g)	**TARGET DOSE:** 4 mg CBD | 0.3 mg THC per tablespoon
EQUIPMENT Blender Measuring spoons One 8-ounce (240-ml) sterilized Mason jar **2½ tablespoons (35 ml) liquified CBD Coconut Oil (page 63)** **1 cup (340 g) honey**	Add the liquified CBD coconut oil and honey into a blender. Blend on high speed for a couple of minutes, then empty the infused honey into a Mason jar. Let your CBD honey settle and give it a good stir before serving. If separation occurs over time, re-emulsify by blending the honey again.

NOTE

By using coconut oil made from CBD flower, your dose per serving size will be lower than the hemp oil honey because it's less concentrated. One tablespoon of CBD Coconut Oil (page 63) is equal to 28 mg CBD/2 mg THC, but your final milligrams will be different depending on your specific source material.

CBD HEMP OIL HONEY

YIELD: 1 cup (340 g)	**TARGET DOSE:** about 16 mg CBD per tablespoon (21 g)
½ tablespoon (8 ml) unflavored hemp CBD oil of your choice (250 mg CBD or your preferred dose) **1 cup (340 g) honey**	Add the hemp CBD oil and honey to a blender. Blend on high speed for a couple of minutes, then empty the infused honey into a Mason jar. Let your CBD honey settle and give it a good stir before serving. If separation occurs over time, re-emulsify by blending the honey again.

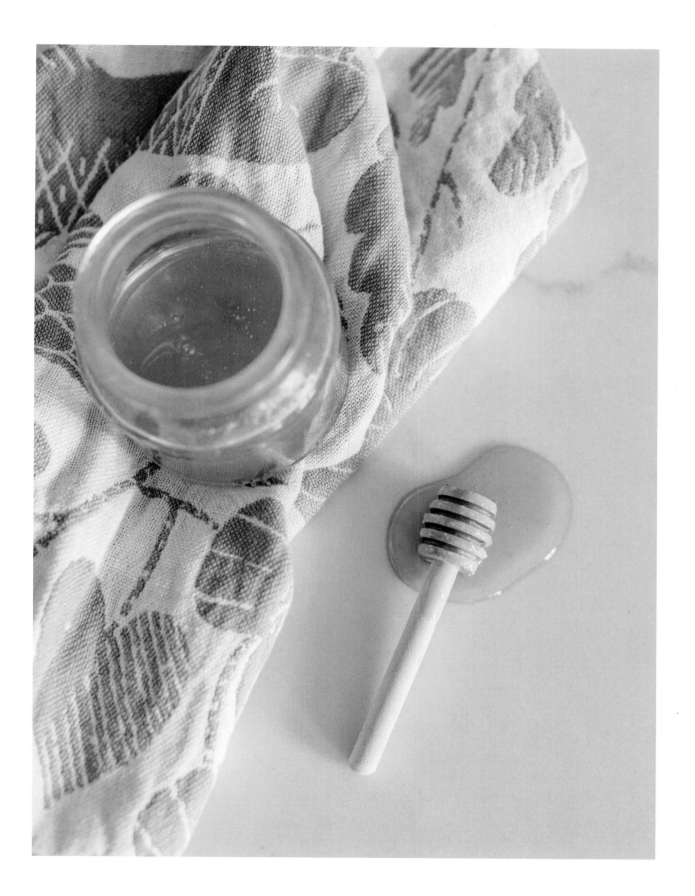

CBD MINT AGAVE SIMPLE SYRUP

If you are planning on making CBD mocktails or cocktails, having an infused simple syrup on hand is a must. You'll find this recipe is easy to infuse with different herbs and spices, if you want to try something other than mint. This CBD simple syrup will be used to infuse Strawberry Mint Agave CBD Iced Tea on page 135, but feel free to add it to a number of different beverages for your enjoyment.

YIELD: 15 ounces (444 ml)	**TARGET DOSE:** 13 mg CBD | 1 mg THC per ounce (30 ml) (using CBD-rich flower method) or 17 mg CBD per ounce (30 ml) (using CBD isolate)

EQUIPMENT
Digital scale
Measuring cups
Measuring spoons
Small saucepan
Thermometer
One 16-ounce (480-ml) sterilized
    Mason jar
Cheesecloth
Fine-mesh strainer

**2 grams decarboxylated CBD-rich
    flower (see note)**
2 cups (480 ml) water
**1 cup (340 g) golden light agave
    nectar**
1 cup (96 g) fresh mint leaves
**1 tablespoon (15 ml) food-grade
    vegetable glycerin**

Weigh out 2 grams of decarboxylated CBD-rich flower. Set aside. Combine the water and agave nectar in a small saucepan. Massage the mint leaves with your hands to release the oils and then add to the saucepan. Bring to a soft boil, stirring until the agave nectar dissolves into the water. Reduce the heat to around 160°F to 180°F (71°C to 82°C) and add the decarboxylated cannabis. Simmer on low for 50 minutes stirring from time to time.

Reduce the heat and add the vegetable glycerin—this will give the CBD and THC something to bind to. Continue to heat and stir for another 10 minutes. Remove from the heat.

Pour the simple syrup into the Mason jar through cheesecloth placed in a fine-mesh strainer. Let cool and shake before serving. Store in the refrigerator for up to 2 weeks.

NOTE

If you don't have access to CBD-rich flower, you can infuse this recipe using CBD isolate powder. Combine the water, agave nectar, and mint leaves in a small saucepan. Bring to a boil, stirring until the agave nectar dissolves. Boil for 1 minute and then reduce the heat. Continue stirring for another 5 minutes. Remove from the heat. Let the simple syrup steep for about 30 minutes to extract the mint oil. Using a fine-mesh strainer and Mason jar, strain the mint leaves from the simple syrup. Once you're done, pour the mint simple syrup back into a small saucepan and begin to heat again. Add the vegetable glycerin and 0.25 grams of CBD isolate powder. Once the mint simple syrup reaches 140°F to 150°F (60°C to 66°C), the CBD isolate powder should begin to melt. Continue to stir for 5 to 10 minutes, then remove from the heat. Let cool and transfer into an airtight Mason jar for storage.

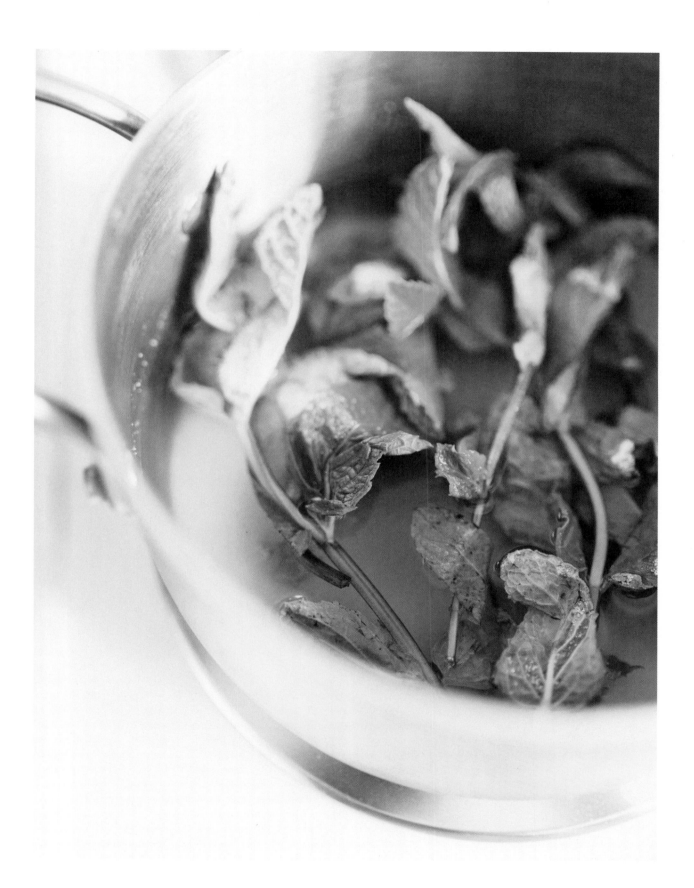

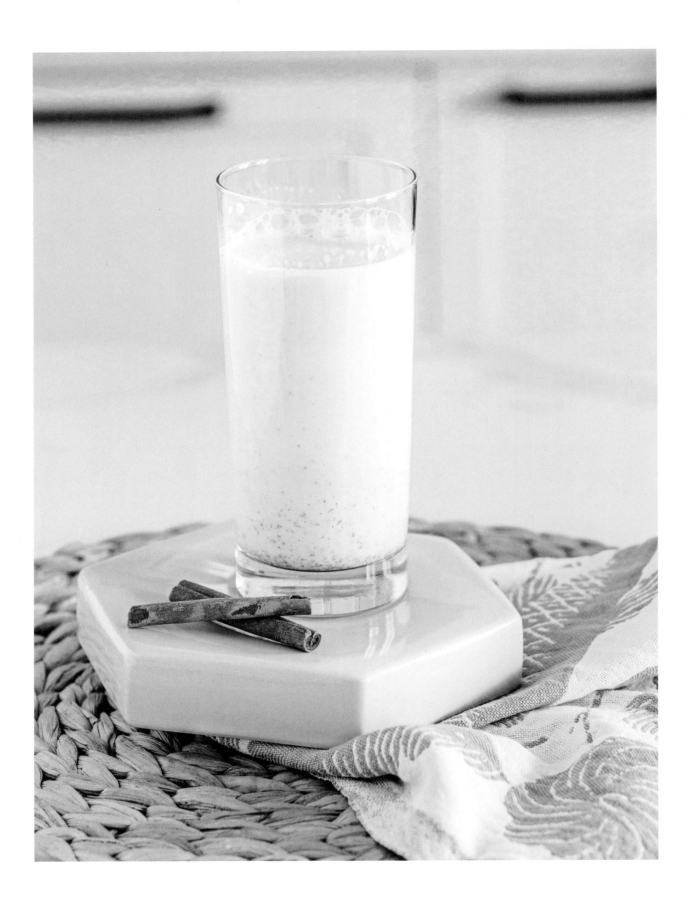

CBD CINNAMON-SPICED MILK

If you love milk in your coffee or tea, this recipe is for you. Full-fat dairy milk and coconut milk are the perfect liquids to extract CBD and THC because of the higher fat content that they present. The higher the fat, the more effective your base solution will be at absorbing the active ingredients that are found in hemp or cannabis. This recipe also includes cinnamon, which contains high amounts of the terpene beta-Caryophyllene. Please note that the final number of servings may vary. If you prefer THC over CBD, try infusing this recipe with THC-rich flower by following the instructions below. Turn to page 132 to use this milk in Hot and Cold CBD Cinnamon-Spiced Coffee.

YIELD: about 23 to 24 ounces (680 to 720 ml)	**TARGET DOSE:** 15 mg CBD	1 mg THC per ounce (30 ml) (using CBD-rich flower method) or 17 mg CBD per ounce (30 ml) (using CBD isolate)

EQUIPMENT

Scale
Measuring cups
Measuring spoons
Small saucepan
Thermometer
Cheesecloth
Fine-mesh strainer
One 24-ounce (720-ml) sterilized
    Mason jar

3.5 grams CBD-rich decarboxylated cannabis flower (see note)

3 cups (720 ml) whole milk (or substitute coconut milk or soymilk)

2 teaspoons (26 g) organic cane sugar

1 teaspoon coconut extract

¼ teaspoon ground cinnamon

Weigh out 3.5 grams of decarboxylated CBD-rich flower. Set aside. Add the milk, sugar, coconut extract, and cinnamon to a saucepan. Bring to a light simmer.

Add the CBD-rich cannabis and keep on low heat (around 160°F, or 71°C). Stir frequently to break up the film on top and scrape the sides to remove cinnamon deposits.

After 1 hour of cooking, remove the infused milk from the heat. Some of the milk will evaporate, so you will have less than your original 3 cups (720 ml).

Using a cheesecloth and fine-mesh strainer, strain the infused milk into a Mason jar for storage. Shake the Mason jar to mix. Let cool and then put in the fridge to chill before serving. If you are not a fan of dairy milk, you can use coconut or soymilk for this infusion. The CBD Cinnamon–Spiced Milk is best if used within a week.

NOTE

If you don't have access to CBD-rich flower to make this infusion, you can still infuse the milk using CBD isolate powder. In a small saucepan, add the milk, sugar, coconut extract, and cinnamon. Heat on low and slowly stir for about 5 to 10 minutes. When the mixture reaches 140°F to 150°F (60°C to 66°C), add 0.40 grams of CBD isolate powder and continue to stir over low heat. Your CBD isolate powder should melt at this point, but be careful the milk never reaches a boil. Continue to stir for another 10 to 15 minutes. Remove from the heat and empty the CBD-infused cinnamon-spiced milk into a Mason jar for storage. Top with an extra dash of cinnamon and shake the Mason jar to mix. Let cool and then put in the fridge to chill before serving.

CBD MATCHA LATTE

Creamy, cozy, and packed with antioxidants, this CBD Matcha Latte is one of my all-time favorites. If you are new to matcha, which means "powdered tea," is it a finely ground powder made of green tea leaves that dissolves instantly in hot water to make warm beverages or it can be used as an exotic flavoring ingredient. Matcha can have a bitter flavor and adding a slight hint of sweetness will provide balance. For this recipe, you'll want to use your CBD Honey (page 124). I also love using coconut or oat milk, but you can easily substitute almond or dairy milk.

YIELD: **1** serving	**TARGET DOSE:** 4 mg CBD | 0.3 mg THC per latte (using DIY CBD Coconut Oil Honey, page 124) or 16 mg CBD per latte (using CBD Hemp Oil Honey, page 124)

EQUIPMENT
One 12-ounce (355-ml) cappuccino cup
Milk frother

1½ teaspoons (3 g) matcha powder (reserve a dash for garnish)

1 tablespoon (15 ml) hot water

1 tablespoon (21 g) CBD honey of your choice (page 124; see note)

1½ cups (360 ml) warmed milk of your choice, frothed

Dash matcha powder

Empty the matcha powder into the cappuccino cup. Add the hot water and CBD honey, and whisk until no matcha powder lumps remain.

If you don't have access to a milk frother, warm the milk and mix it into the other ingredients. Or, using a milk frother, froth or warm the milk and pour on top of your serving cup—latte art not required but if you can pull it off, bravo! Sprinkle a dash of matcha powder on top for garnish.

This matcha latte can also be made cold. Simply follow the directions above, but add the ingredients to a Mason jar, top with cold milk of your choice, seal, and shake vigorously to combine. Serve over ice.

NOTE

If you don't have time to make CBD-infused honey, you can still incorporate CBD into this recipe by adding your favorite full-spectrum hemp CBD oil (at your preferred dose) by whisking it into the matcha powder, water, and honey before adding the milk. Because you are using an oil, separation will occur, but do your best to stir in the CBD oil evenly.

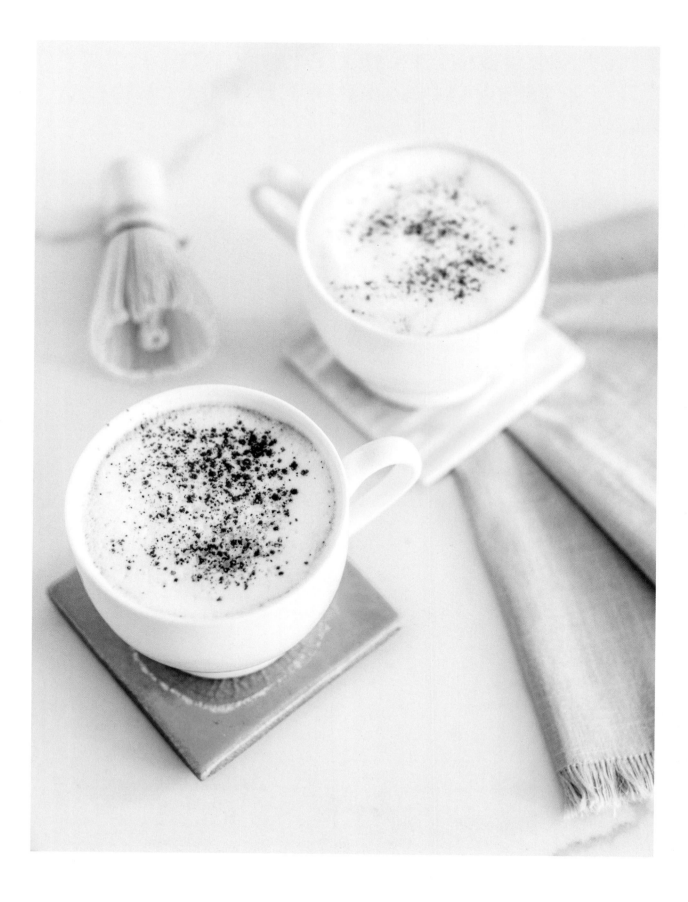

HOT AND COLD CBD CINNAMON-SPICED COFFEE

If you're like me, you're a big fan of hot coffee and cold coffee. Whether you're nestled up with a warm cup of joe or sipping a refreshing cold brew during the peak of summer, there's always a time and place to enjoy both. Infusing pure coffee with CBD can be tricky. This recipe incorporates the CBD cinnamon-spiced milk infusion that you've already created, along with a delicious blend of cinnamon and nutmeg flavors.

HOT CBD CINNAMON-SPICED COFFEE

YIELD: **1** serving	**TARGET DOSE:** 15 mg CBD | 1 mg THC per coffee (using DIY CBD Cinnamon-Spiced Milk, page 129) or 17 mg CBD per coffee (using commercially made CBD oil or tincture, see note below)

EQUIPMENT
Coffee maker
Milk frother
Standard coffee cup

CINNAMON- NUTMEG COFFEE

4 to 5 tablespoons (12 to 15 g) ground coffee (+/- if you prefer weaker/ stronger coffee)

1 teaspoon ground cinnamon

1 teaspoon ground nutmeg

4 cups (960 ml) water

HOT CBD COFFEE

1 ounce (30 ml) CBD Cinnamon-Spiced Milk (page 129), frothed

1 ounce (30 ml) milk of your choice, frothed

6 ounces (177 ml) hot coffee

Sprinkle ground cinnamon, nutmeg, and organic sugar (optional)

To make the cinnamon-nutmeg coffee, combine the ground coffee, cinnamon, and nutmeg in the filter of a coffee maker. Add the water and turn on the coffee maker to brew.

To make the hot CBD coffee, using a milk frother, combine the cinnamon-spiced milk with regular milk and froth.

When your coffee is done brewing, pour the coffee into a standard coffee cup and top with frothed milk. Add a dash of cinnamon, nutmeg, and sugar on top (if using). Save the leftover brewed coffee and chill to make iced coffee drinks.

NOTE

If you didn't have time to make the CBD-infused cinnamon-spiced milk and still want to add commercially made CBD oil into this recipe, simply add ½ dropper of your favorite unflavored CBD oil at 17 milligrams (or your pre-ferred dose) to the coffee before you add the non-infused frothed milk. Just be aware that oil and liquids do not mix well, so you might have oil drops that float to the top of the drink if you use an oil-based tincture.

COLD CBD CINNAMON-SPICED COFFEE

SERVINGS: 1	TARGET DOSE: 15 mg CBD | 1 mg THC per coffee (using CBD Cinnamon-Spiced Milk, page 129) or 17 mg CBD per coffee (using commercially made CBD oil, see note below)

EQUIPMENT
Collins glass
Spoon for stirring

½ cup ice

12 to 16 ounces (355 to 473 ml) chilled Cinnamon-Nutmeg Coffee (opposite)

1 ounce (30 ml) CBD Cinnamon-Spiced Milk (page 129), plus more to taste

Dash sugar (optional)

Fill a Collins glass with ice and top with chilled coffee. Slowly stir in the CBD cinnamon-spiced milk with a spoon. Add a dash of sugar if you prefer a sweeter taste.

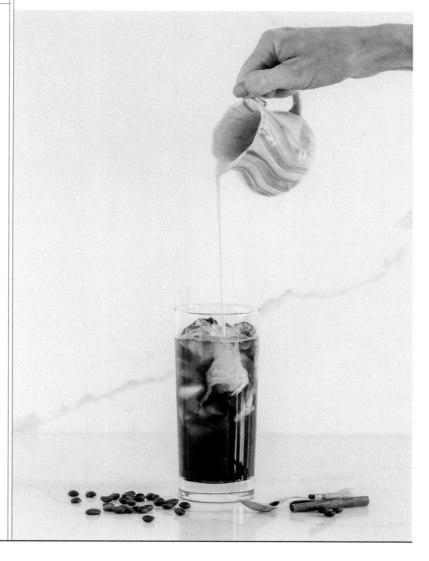

CBD & BEVERAGES

NOTE

If you didn't have time to make the CBD-infused cinnamon-spiced milk and still want to add commercially made CBD oil into this recipe, simply add ½ dropper of your favorite unflavored CBD oil (at 17 milligrams or your preferred dose) into a shaker tin or large Mason jar, add the coffee and non-infused milk, then vigorously shake. Pour on top of a glass of ice and serve as directed.

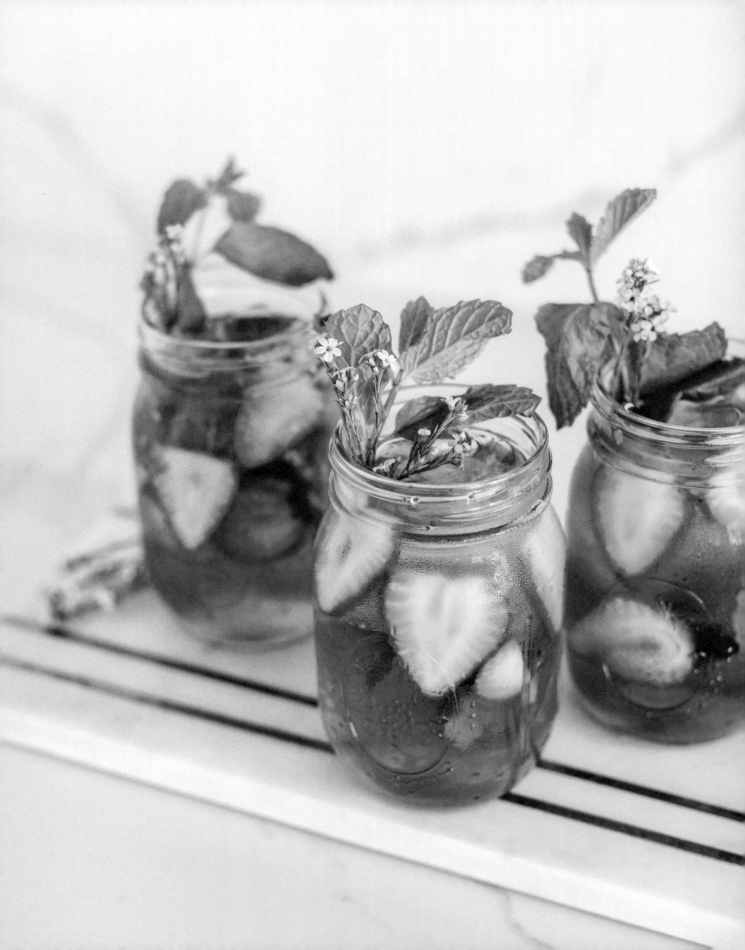

STRAWBERRY MINT AGAVE
CBD ICED TEA

There's nothing better than a glass of cold iced tea on a hot day. The CBD Mint Agave Simple Syrup (page 126) that you've already created is the perfect match for the other refreshing ingredients that are used in this recipe. By incorporating fresh strawberries and mint, this thirst-quenching beverage not only looks and tastes great, but it's packed with healing benefits!

YIELD: 1 serving	**TARGET DOSE:** 13 mg CBD	1 mg THC per tea (using CBD Mint Agave Simple Syrup, page 126) or 17 mg CBD per tea (using commercially made CBD oil or tincture, see note below)

EQUIPMENT
Collins glass or Mason jar
Muddler

8 to 10 fresh mint leaves (plus a small sprig for garnish)

2 large strawberries, sliced (plus a few slices for serving)

1 ounce (30 ml) CBD Mint Agave Simple Syrup (page 126; plus more if you prefer sweeter; see note)

1 cup ice

12 to 16 ounces (355 to 473 ml) mint iced tea

Place the mint leaves, strawberries, and simple syrup in a glass. Muddle the ingredients to release the strawberry juices and mint oils. By muddling, you are also integrating the CBD into your other ingredients.

Add ice and pour the mint iced tea on top. Stir to mix all ingredients. Line the inside of a Collins glass or Mason jar with berry slices.

Serve the iced tea in the glass garnished with a sprig of mint and a slice of strawberry.

For this recipe, I used spearmint-peppermint herbal tea to make the iced tea (1 tea bag per cup).

NOTE

If you don't have the supplies to make the CBD Mint Agave Simple Syrup, substitute regular simple syrup and add ½ dropper of your favorite unflavored CBD oil (at 17 milligrams or your preferred dose) to the glass before muddling. After this step, proceed with the recipe as noted and enjoy.

TROPICAL GINGER TURMERIC CBD SMOOTHIE

I just can't get enough of this delicious smoothie. Combining exotic flavors of tropical fruits plus a super blend of ginger and turmeric, this smoothie will brighten your day with its powerful antioxidant properties. This healing combination fights inflammation, helps with digestion, and can boost your immune system. When combined with CBD, this smoothie is just what the doctor ordered.

YIELD: 1 serving	**TARGET DOSE:** 4 mg CBD | 0.3 mg THC per smoothie (using DIY CBD Coconut Oil Honey, page 124) or 16 mg CBD per smoothie (using CBD Hemp Oil Honey, page 124)

EQUIPMENT
Blender
One 17-ounce (503-ml) stemless wine
    glass

Add the banana, strawberries, pineapple, orange juice, yogurt, CBD honey, chia seeds, turmeric, and ginger to a blender. Blend until smooth and creamy.

Serve in the wine glass topped with a slice of pineapple.

1 banana

½ cup (127 g) frozen strawberries

½ cup (85 g) fresh pineapple chunks

½ cup (120 ml) fresh orange juice (adjust down if you prefer a thicker smoothie)

1 tablespoon (15 g) coconut milk yogurt (nondairy preferred)

1 tablespoon (21 g) CBD honey of your choice (adjust down if you prefer; see note)

1 teaspoon chia seeds

¼ teaspoon ground turmeric

¼ teaspoon ground ginger

1 slice pineapple, for garnish

NOTE

If you don't have time to make CBD-infused honey, you can still incorporate CBD into this recipe by adding your favorite unflavored CBD oil (at your preferred dose) into the blender. Simply blend with the other ingredients and enjoy.

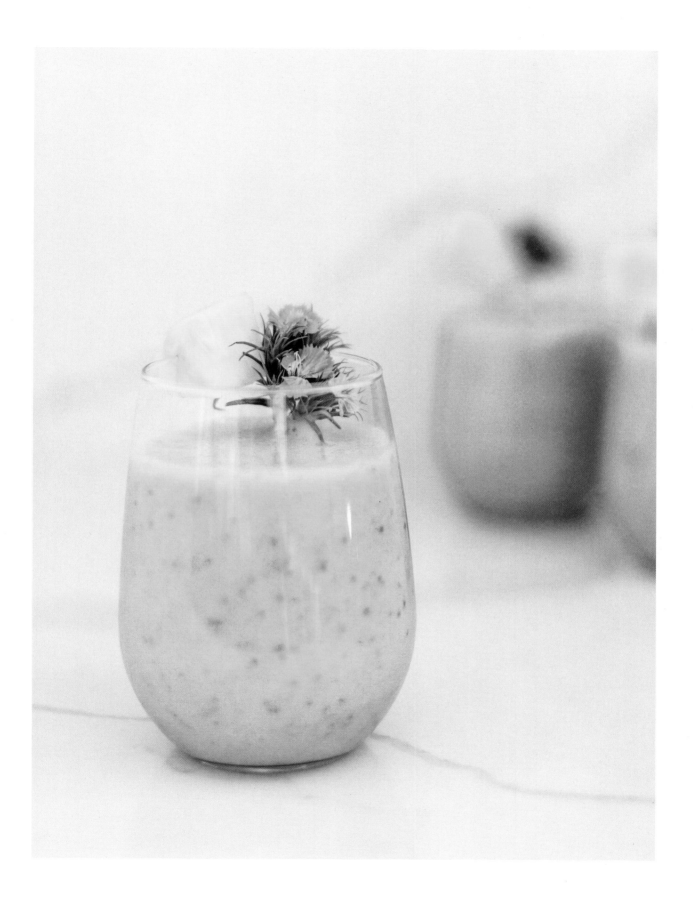

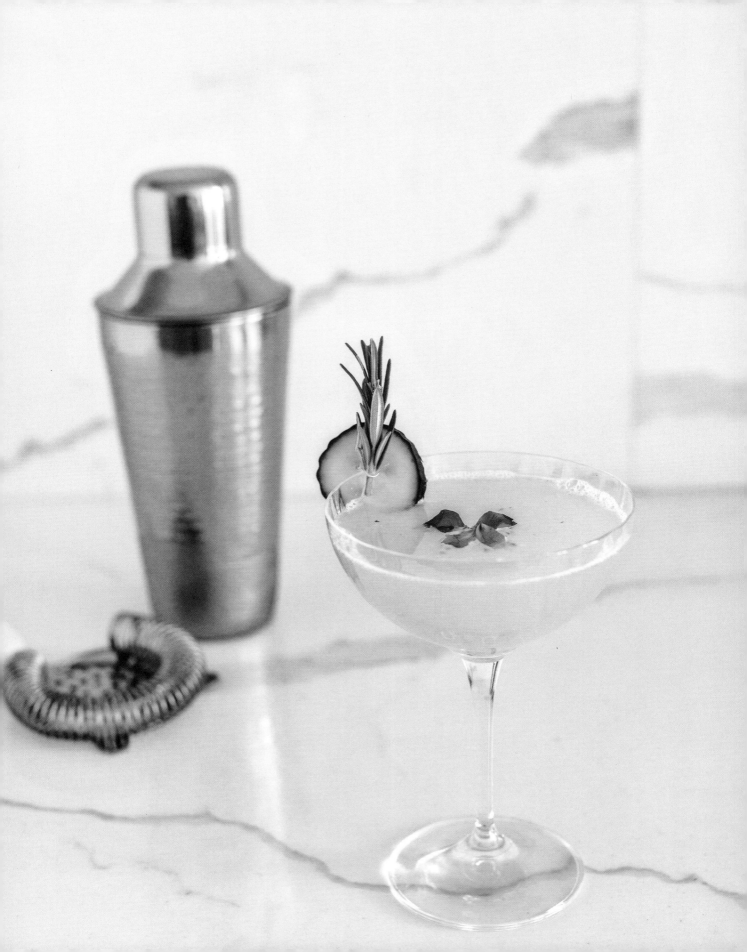

ROSEMARY CUCUMBER CBD GIMLET

crafted by Rachel Burkons of Altered Plates

Looking to impress your friends with a gorgeous infused drink? Rachel Burkons has created a perfect recipe that combines the tantalizing flavors of rosemary, rosewater, cucumber, and lime juice. This refreshing CBD drink is always a hit at parties. You can serve it as a mocktail or easily convert it to a cocktail by using a nice botanical gin.

YIELD: **1** serving

TARGET DOSE:
17 mg CBD (using a commercially made CBD oil or tincture)

EQUIPMENT
Muddler
Shaker tin
Strainer
Coupe glass

3 rosemary sprigs, divided

4 thick slices English cucumber, divided

1 ounce (30 ml) fresh lime juice

½ teaspoon rosewater

½ dropper CBD tincture of your choice (17 mg CBD or your preferred dose)

¾ ounce (22 ml) simple syrup

2 ounces (60 ml) gin (optional)

Ice, for shaking

Soda water, for topping

Destem two of the rosemary sprigs. In a shaker tin, muddle the destemmed rosemary and three slices of the cucumber until fragrant. Add the lime juice, rosewater, CBD tincture, simple syrup, and gin (if using). Add ice and shake for 10 seconds. Strain and serve in a coupe glass.

Top with soda water; garnish with a rosemary sprig and a cucumber slice.

CBD OLD-FASHIONED

crafted by John Korkidis of *Chron Vivant*

John Korkidis: "Few cocktails have stood the test of time like the old-fashioned and knowing how to craft a proper one is a staple in the repertoire of any 'Chron Vivant.' One of my personal favorites, this timeless libation can be elevated with a dash of CBD bitters for a nightcap that's sure to soothe any weary soul. Though it's not the 'oldest' cocktail, it is closest to the original definition of the word (bitters, spirits, sugar, and water). These days you can even find cannabis-inspired versions of this concoction popping up at bars and underground supper clubs, where experts in the craft are coming up with their own creative spin.

The simplicity of an old-fashioned naturally lends itself to interpretation and even though there really is no wrong way to build this modern classic, one thing is for certain: It must contain bitters. In this case, you're using your homemade CBD bitters recipe (page 113) that pairs perfectly with brown spirits such as bourbon and rye. This 'house' bitter contains a broad-spectrum CBD so there will be trace amounts of other compounds and terpenes to help modulate mild relaxing effects. Below is my recipe for a classic old-fashioned bourbon whiskey cocktail with a modern CBD twist."

YIELD: **1** serving	**TARGET DOSE:** 5 mg CBD (using DIY CBD Bitters, page 113)

EQUIPMENT
Whiskey glass
Bar spoon

Ice cube, for serving

2 ounces (60 ml) rye or bourbon whiskey (we'll be using bourbon)

¼ ounce (7 ml) simple syrup (The 1880 recipe calls for a sugar cube, but most modern recipes call for simple syrup as it easily dissolves making for a cleaner drink.)

2 dashes Angostura bitters

1 dash Chron Vivant CBD Bitters (page 113; see note)

Lemon twist, for garnish

Fill an old-fashioned whiskey glass with a singular ice cube (neither too large nor too small). Pour rye or bourbon over the ice. Add the simple syrup, bitters, and stir. Finally, express the oils from the lemon peel and garnish. (The essence of the lemon can be extracted by breaking the delicate vessels that contain high concentrations of limonene terpenes and other mood-enhancing aromatics.)

The end result should be mildly sweet and strong, but always balanced. Neither the cannabis bitters, syrup, nor the spirit, should be dominant over the other. Have fun mixing and matching spirits and bitters, and enjoy for the relaxing effects and also the flavor and aromas that pair well together.

NOTE

If you don't have the materials to make CBD bitters, you can still incorporate CBD into this recipe by adding your favorite unflavored CBD tincture (at your preferred dose) into the drink. Simply add the CBD to the glass, top with the other ingredients, stir vigorously with a spoon, and serve. Just be aware that separation will occur if you are using an oil-based CBD tincture.

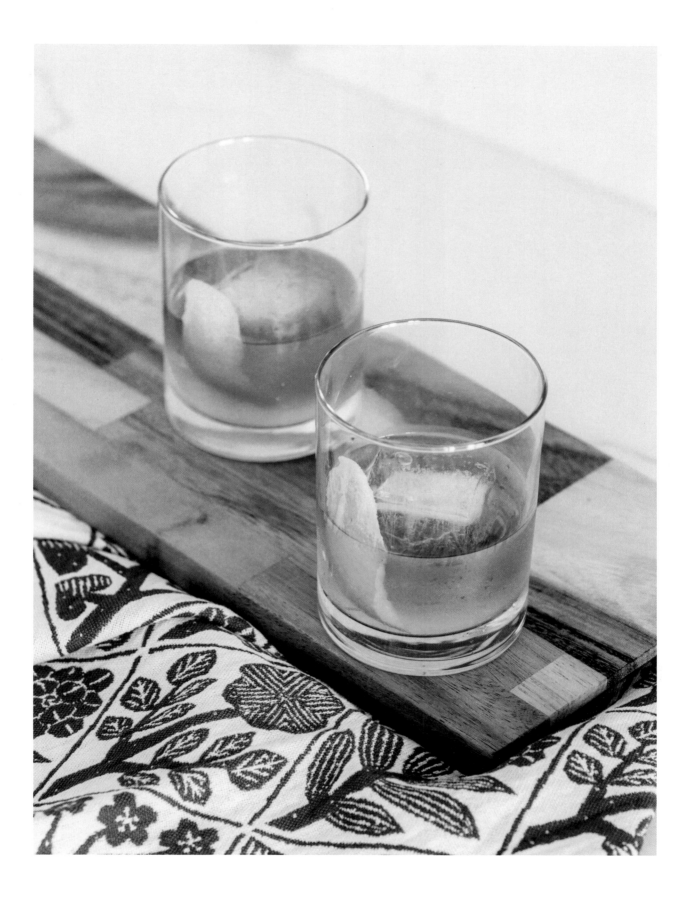

THE PERFECT CBD COCKTAIL

Q&A *with* Warren Bobrow, The Cocktail Whisperer & author of *Cannabis Cocktails, Mocktails & Tonics*

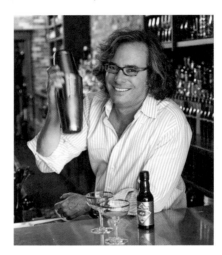

Warren Bobrow, The Cocktail Whisperer, is the multi-published author of Apothecary Cocktails; Whiskey Cocktails; Bitters and Shrub Syrup Cocktails; Cannabis Cocktails, Mocktails & Tonics; *and his celebrated 2017 release,* The Craft Cocktail Compendium. *Warren has written articles for* Saveur *magazine,* Voda *magazine,* Whole Foods *Dark Rye,* Distiller, Beverage Media, DrinkupNY, *and many other national and global periodicals. Follow his cocktail adventures on Twitter @WarrenBobrow1 or Instagram @warrenbobrow.*

Q: What are three facts every beginner should know when making infused cocktails at home?

A: "Start slow. Always decarb. Remember the Thai food principal, don't make it too spicy right away."

Q: What do you consider a standard dose for a single serving of a CBD-infused cocktail?

A: "If you're using a tincture, start with ten drops of your favorite CBD product or start with your desired dose. Build up from there. Alcohol really negates CBD, so it's probably not the most efficient way to consume it if you're looking for maximum therapeutic effects."

Q: When combining CBD with alcohol, what are some precautions a beginner should be aware of?

A: "CBD is pretty innocuous stuff. There really aren't any warnings. Just experiment on yourself to find the right balance. Don't worry, you won't get high! To experiment with CBD cocktails on your own, I've put together a special Roasted CBD Citrus Punch recipe for you to try at home."

ROASTED CBD CITRUS PUNCH

YIELD: 6 to 8 servings	TARGET DOSE: your choice (using commercially made CBD oil or tincture)

EQUIPMENT
Baking pan
Citrus juicer
Double jigger

4 ounces (115 g) orange

4 ounces (115 g) grapefruit

4 ounces (115 g) pomelo

4 ounces (115 g) tangerine

Dash of Angostura bitters

Demerara sugar (optional)

3 ounces (89 ml) Fruitations simple syrup of tangerine (I used this simple syrup for balance)

750 milliliters (1 bottle) ginger ale (cane sugar over corn syrup)

Pinch sea salt

Dash cardamom bitters

Dash chocolate mole bitters

CBD oil of your choice (your desired dose)

Splash rhum agricole (optional)

Preheat the oven to 300°F (150°C). Halve the citrus and roast with Angostura bitters and a sprinkle of Demerara sugar (if using). Let cool and then juice.

Combine all the roasted juices, simple syrup, and ginger ale in a punch bowl. Add a good pinch of sea salt. Add the bitters, dot with CBD, and add a splash of rhum agricole (if using). How much? About that much. Stir and serve.

143

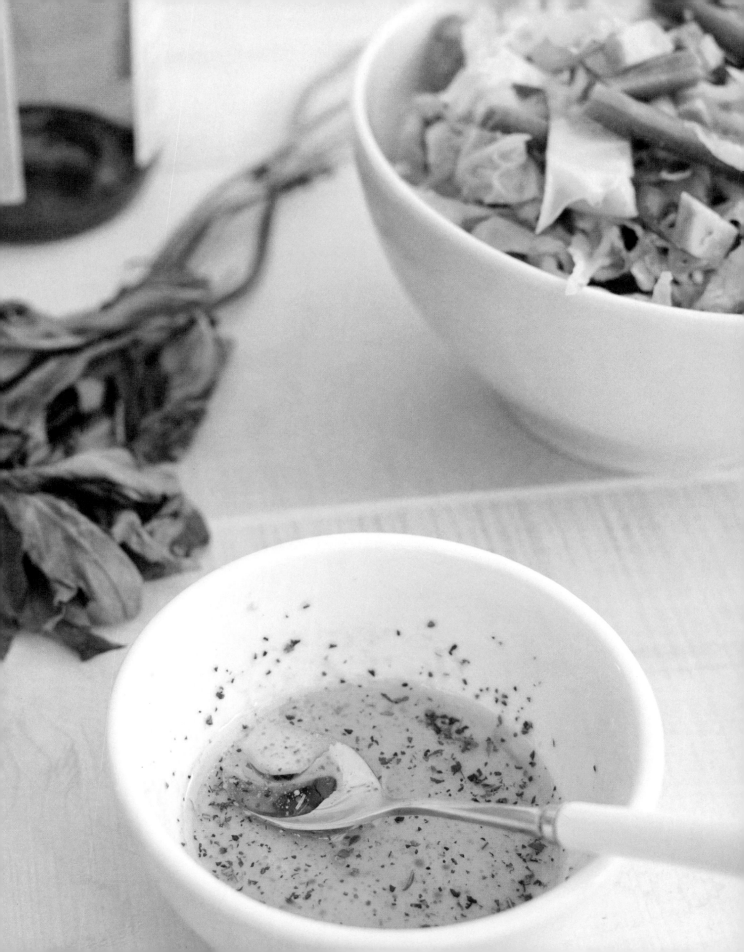

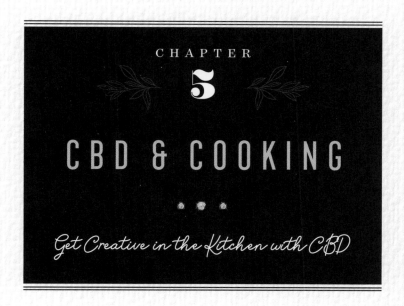

CHAPTER

5

CBD & COOKING

• • •

Get Creative in the Kitchen with CBD

There's nothing better than sharing a delicious meal with family and friends. Food is what brings us together. From sourcing the perfect ingredients to creating thoughtful pairings and finding the perfect sauce to complement a dish, there's an art to cooking and crafting an unforgettable dining experience.

While there are many components to a recipe that help create the finest fare, chefs across the nation are particularly excited about a few new ingredient options. Dining is not just about food and wine anymore. Cannabis has opened the door to a new world of aromas, flavors, and effects that can be integrated into a menu.

Professional chefs aren't the only ones finding pleasure in experimenting with CBD, THC, and terpenes. If you're a passionate foodie or at-home chef, you can easily integrate elevated ingredients into your favorite recipes as long as you know the basics when it comes to cooking with cannabis- and hemp-derived products.

As any chef would agree, there is endless potential when it comes to infusing cuisine. You can be as creative as you want to be as long as you learn an effective, consistent, and safe method of working with the material. Cannabis has the ability to enhance flavors and enhance euphoria, adding an entirely new dynamic to the dining experience.

By learning the ins and outs, you'll be able to craft delicious infused cuisine at home. Master the art of infusions, explore CBD-rich flower and food pairings, plus prepare a variety of DIY recipes to share with your friends. It's time to put your chef hat on and get cooking!

INFUSED FOODS 101

Infused food refers to edible products or cuisine that has been infused with CBD, THC, or other plant-based compounds and materials. When cooking, you can use both cannabis or hemp to enhance a variety of recipes, which typically begins by creating an oil- or butter-based infusion. Think of these as your "pantry items" that you will then use in your final dishes.

As you will learn, you can create these infusions by using cannabis flower or isolate; however, if you have access to CBD-rich flower, by all means, I recommend using it in your recipes. You can also substitute professionally made full-spectrum hemp CBD oil into your recipes, if you don't have the time to make your own.

Whatever method you decide to use, cooking infused food takes practice and patience. If you're planning to cook for others, it's essential to learn the dos and don'ts to ensure a safe and responsible meal. As an at-home chef, handling cannabis with the utmost care should be your number one priority. Plus, you should fully understand how edibles differ from other forms of cannabis and hemp products, so there are no surprises after consuming them.

ENJOYING INFUSED FOODS SAFELY & RESPONSIBLY

Before making your first infused dish, it's imperative to educate yourself on edibles and understand how your body will react after consuming them. Many people believe that eating an edible is the same as smoking CBD or THC, but as you've learned in the last chapter (see page 101), this is not true. Most importantly, remember that having a high tolerance when smoking/vaping does not mean you'll have the same tolerance with edibles.

After consuming CBD- or THC-infused foods, effects typically kick in within 1 to 2 hours depending on your metabolism, body weight, endocannabinoid system, what else you've eaten, plus many other factors. Just like CBD beverages, CBD-infused foods won't get you high, but THC foods will. Depending on the amount of THC you've consumed, effects can linger for up to 8 hours or longer. You should always strategically plan on when you'll eat THC-infused edibles or cuisine to ensure that you have the best experience possible.

While CBD effects are more subtle, it is very easy to overdo it with THC if you're not patient. If you don't feel the effects right away, do not eat more. Overindulging is, unfortunately, a lesson many of us have learned the hard way.

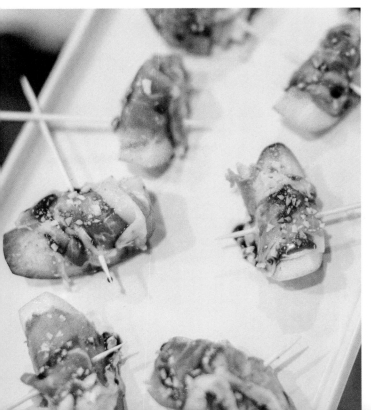

Left: Chef Coreen Carroll's Serrano Ham and Peaches drizzled with CBD sugar beet syrup served at an Herb Somm event.

Opposite: For formal infused dining events, impress your guests with a beautifully set table including a printed menu and other educational materials that might help guide the elevated experience.

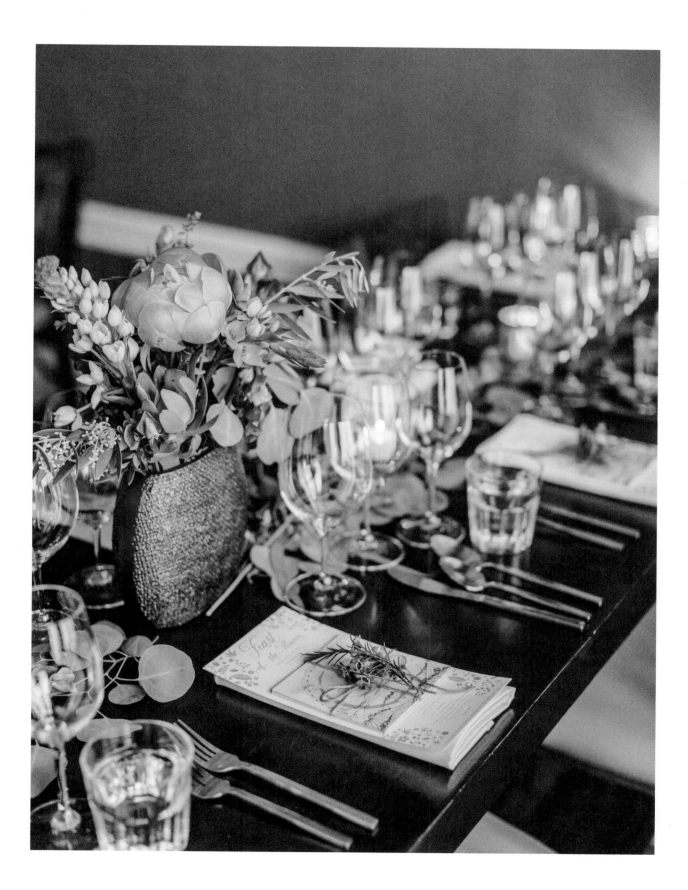

If you are using THC edibles or infused foods for sleep, a trick that I've learned is to not eat them right before bed. If you do, effects will hit your body in the middle of the night, which can disrupt the sleep cycle or cause an edible "hangover" in the morning. Unlike an alcohol hangover, you won't feel sick from edibles, but you might feel really tired and groggy the next morning if you eat them too late. From personal experience, to achieve best results, consume infused foods or edibles at least 1½ to 2 hours before sleeping.

CBD edibles or foods could have the opposite effect depending on what product you are using. For instance, I've mistakenly eaten an uplifting CBD gummy before bed and couldn't fall asleep if my life depended on it! Get to know your products well before using them. Be smart, consume responsibly, and remember the golden rule to any edible or infused cuisine experience, "start low, go slow."

COOKING WITH CANNABIS & HEMP PRODUCTS

Like many other herbs, cannabis is a food-friendly plant that is full of aromas, flavors, and nutrition. To cook with it properly, there are several techniques that you can use to ensure your infused foods turn out well after baking, mixing, heating, etc.

Chef Coreen Carroll, a professional cannabis chef and co-founder of the Cannaisseur Series in San Francisco, explains that the major difference between cooking with THC versus CBD is the intoxicating effects. Yet, when it comes down to technique the same rules apply for both. Below is a five-step checklist every beginner should know before stepping foot in the kitchen.

CHOOSE THE RIGHT STRAIN OR PRODUCT

The first step to creating infused foods is selecting the correct strain or product that will be used in the recipe. If you're making a CBD-rich flower infusion, the best piece of advice I can give is to smell a selection of different strains, if possible, to see what type of flower smells best to you. This is usually an indication of what terpenes your body is craving—your nose knows!

When selecting a strain, it's also important to consider how you want to feel. What effect are you trying to achieve? Remember, it isn't just about looking for "sativa" or "indica." To find the best product, it is important to understand the strain's terpene profile and consider the entourage effect of THC, CBD, THCA, and other cannabinoids that are present.

Chef Coreen Carroll also notes that quality infusions start with quality material. You can really taste the difference between an infused good that was made with high-quality flower versus old, dry, or stale material.

Once you select a strain, make a note of the pronounced aromas and flavors, plus cannabinoid percentages that are listed on the packaging, then do your dosage calculations to best estimate final CBD and THC per serving (see calculations on page 52). It's incredibly hard to accurately measure dosages in infused beverages and cuisine, so do your best, stick to one strain per infusion, and serve responsibly.

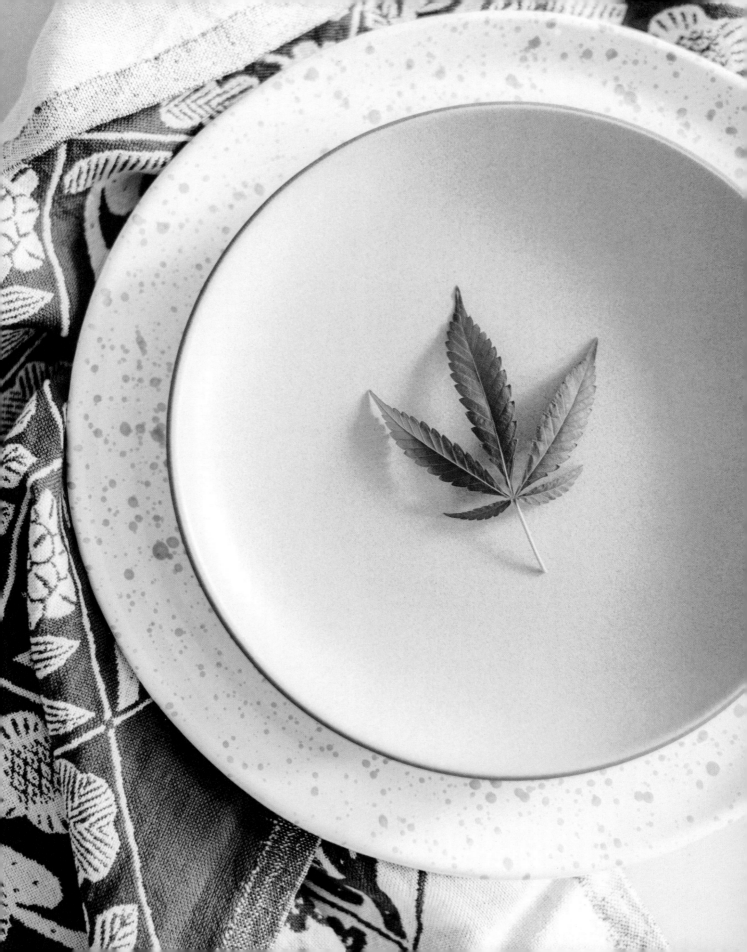

If you don't plan to use CBD-rich flower in your infusion, there are many other professionally made products that you can use in your recipe. CBD oils, CBD honey, and CBD cooking powders are all great options. Before integrating it into a recipe, make sure to taste the product so you know how the flavors will interact with your other ingredients and, above all, figure out the proper dosages before you start cooking.

CHOOSE YOUR INGREDIENTS

Now that you know what CBD material you'd like to use in your recipe, it's time to think about the ingredients that you'll be cooking with. Will the flavors work with the strain or product you've selected?

As you might have encountered, at-home infusions and professionally made items can often have a green taste to them. Some chefs are experts at masking herbaceous flavors, while others like to enhance cannabis and hemp's natural characteristics by using complementary ingredients (see page 157 for a list of suggestions). Trust your palate on what flavor combinations work best. As you will learn, mastering flavor pairings takes practice, but it's incredibly fun.

DECARBOXYLATE, DECARBOXYLATE, DECARBOXYLATE!

The number one rookie mistake made when cooking is forgetting to decarboxylate your cannabis or hemp flower. If you want more intense and enhanced effects, decarbing is your best option (see page 48). Activation for high CBD strains begins between 240°F and 295°F (115°C–146°C) for 20 to 60 minutes and between 240°F and 275°F (115°C–135°C) for 20 to 60 minutes for THC dominant strains.

The decarboxylation method that's used in this book is the method that I learned from professional cannabis chef Coreen Carroll of the Cannaisseur Series. She recommends to first set your oven to 275°F (135°C). Next, line a baking sheet with parchment paper or aluminum foil and use your fingers or scissors to cut up your flower into pea-sized pieces. Spread the dry flower evenly across the baking sheet and bake for 20 minutes. No matter what method you choose, stay within the 240°F to 295°F (115°C–146°C) range when decarboxylating and do not exceed 300°F (150°C).

Chef Calvin Eng, a professional chef based in Brooklyn, also recommends using all parts of the flower when decarboxylating, including stems, buds, and shake. Don't waste! Just make sure it's the same strain.

CONSIDER INFUSION OPTIONS

After successfully decarboxylating your product, the next step is creating your infusion. Using a substance that is fat-based to extract CBD (and THC) is one of your best options, especially when mixing with food. In the coming pages, you will learn how to infuse your recipes using CBD butter, olive oil, and coconut oil. You will also learn how to infuse avocado oil with Monica Lo, founder of Sous Weed. If you've purchased a professionally made cannabis or hemp product, most of the hard work has already been done for you. Your task now is to start cooking, using the product as directed.

GET COOKING

The last step on this checklist is to finally make the recipe by incorporating your infusion. Treat the infusion as an ingredient and make sure you have the proper equipment and accessories on hand that allow for accurate measurements. This is the most important part of creating infused cuisine. Know your dosages and measurements!

MIXING CBD INTO YOUR FAVORITE FOODS

There are a number of different ways you can prepare CBD-infused cuisine. For beginners, you'll most often craft an infusion using CBD-rich flower or simply mix professionally made CBD oil into a recipe. You can also use CBD isolate to make an infusion if you have access to a reliable resource. Set aside any alcohol-based tinctures or alcohol-based infusions that you might have created in the last chapter. These aren't the best options for food recipes. Instead, let's review what works best for cuisine.

CBD-RICH FLOWER & CBD ISOLATE INFUSIONS

If you choose to work with CBD-rich flower or CBD isolates, typically mixing these substances with olive oil, coconut oil, butter, or ghee is the perfect combination to elevate any meal. Preparing infused butter, oil, etc., is a fairly simple process, but the techniques for creating the infusion vary. Let's go through each one.

Oil-Based Infusions

Two common oil-based infusions are olive oil and coconut oil. Both of these products are used in many different types of recipes and are extremely easy to work with. Much like finding a good source of CBD, you'll also want to find a quality oil to use in your infusions. For instance, you'll want to avoid olive oils that are grassy, herbaceous, and bitter—while those styles can be great on their own, those characteristics can often be accentuated when combined with cannabis flavors.

I usually have both olive oil and coconut oil options ready to use in my kitchen because they impart different flavors and characteristics to a recipe. For instance, if I am preparing a savory dish that expresses Mediterranean flavors and spices, infused olive oil is what I'll use in the recipe. Because coconut oil is so expressive of coconut flavors, I love adding it to a variety of dessert recipes and honey. Refer back to chapter 2 to learn how to infuse both (see page 61 for olive oil and page 63 for coconut oil).

Butter Infusions

Creating infused butter at home is pretty straightforward. It can be integrated into a variety of recipes and is the perfect ingredient to add to a number of baked goods. Before making an infused butter, head to the grocery store and look for a butter brand that contains higher levels of fat. High-fat butter is the best to use because it'll bind to cannabinoids and other compounds easily, allowing you to get the most out of your infusion. When comparing American versus European butter, the standards for the minimum amount of butterfat in butter vary. American butter is 80 percent fat, whereas European butter has a minimum of 82 percent fat. The higher the fat content, the easier the butter will bind to CBD and other important compounds. I also recommend using unsalted butter, so you can more accurately control the amount of salt that goes into the final recipe. For a butter recipe, see page 64.

FULL-SPECTRUM CBD OIL-BASED TINCTURES

If you don't have time to create your own infusion, you can easily add drops of a professionally made full-spectrum CBD oil into your recipes. If you decide to use this method to infuse cuisine, look for brands that use olive oil as the carrier and try to find an oil that is unflavored so you can taste the other flavors of the ingredients that you are cooking with. You'll also want to set your expensive CBD oil tinctures aside because you might have to use a good portion of the bottle to account for the amount that's called for in a recipe. For example, 1 tablespoon equals about 15 ml. If you have a 30-ml bottle of full-spectrum CBD oil, this would be half of your bottle.

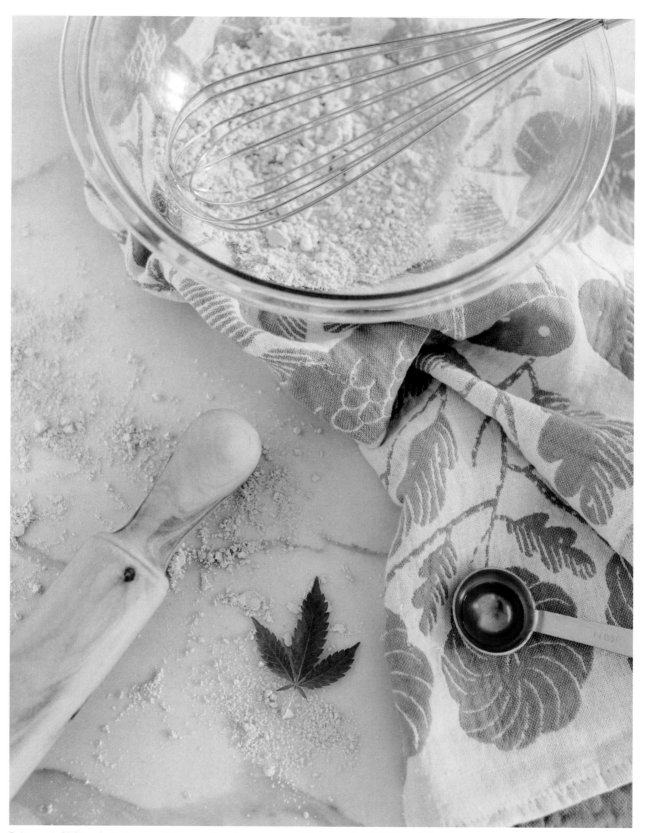

Baking with CBD is a fantastic way to infuse your favorite sweet treats. All you need is CBD-infused oil or butter.

THE SOUS VIDE METHOD

featuring Monica Lo, founder of *Sous Weed*

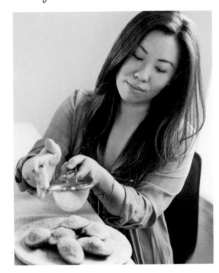

Monica Lo is the founder of Sous Weed, a popular infused cooking and recipe website that teaches readers how to use the sous vide method when cooking with cannabis. In addition to her work in the canna-culinary space, she is also a professional food photographer and creative director working to change public perception of cannabis users. Monica has shot and helped styled the award-winning Sous Vide at Home *cookbook with Penguin Random House as well as the sequel,* Sous Vide Made Simple, *which was released in fall 2018. Follow Monica @sousweed or visit sousweed.com.*

Monica Lo: "At Sous Weed, I use the sous vide method to make cannabis infusions for world-class edibles. For those unfamiliar, sous vide is an increasingly popular cooking technique that calls for sealing your ingredients (in this case, CBD-heavy cannabis flower and your preferred oil) in a vacuum-sealed bag or Mason jar and cooking them in a precise-temperature water bath.

The gentle cooking temperature means that the delicate terpenes will be left intact. Temperature control with a sous vide machine is so precise: that means you won't accidentally burn the flower or the oil creating a bitter, acrid taste that people sometimes associate with a bad pot brownie.

All your delicious recipes can be designed around the different flavor profiles of specific strains so you can make various infusions using different strains. Find a strain with a sweet, fruity terpene profile for desserts versus one that's herbaceous or earthy, which would work better in a savory dish. To try the sous vide method on your own, here is a recipe that I've developed for an infused Sous Weed CBD Avocado Oil. I've also created a Creamy (No Cream!) CBD Sweet Corn Chowder for you to enjoy. See page 181 for the recipe."

SOUS WEED CBD AVOCADO OIL

YIELD: **16** ounces (475 ml) | **TARGET DOSE:** Varies depending on strain (See page 52 to calculate your own dosage.)

EQUIPMENT

Sous vide precision cooker

Two 16-ounce (480-ml) sterilized Mason jars

Large pot (or bath) of water

Tongs

Cheesecloth

Fine-mesh strainer

2 cups (480 ml) avocado oil

½ ounce (15 g) CBD-heavy cannabis flower, roughly broken up

Set your sous vide water bath to 185°F (85°C). Pour the avocado oil into a large Mason jar and add the CBD-heavy cannabis flower. Seal the jar and place it into the water bath to sous vide for 4 hours. Gently remove the jar from the water bath using tongs and let cool.

Prepare the cheesecloth by placing it over the fine-mesh strainer. Strain the infused oil into a clean Mason jar. Keep the oil in a cool dark place or in the fridge.

NOTE

You can choose to decarboxylate your flower before adding it into this recipe by using the method listed in the book (see page 48); however, sometimes I go straight to using the sous vide method to best preserve the terpene profiles.

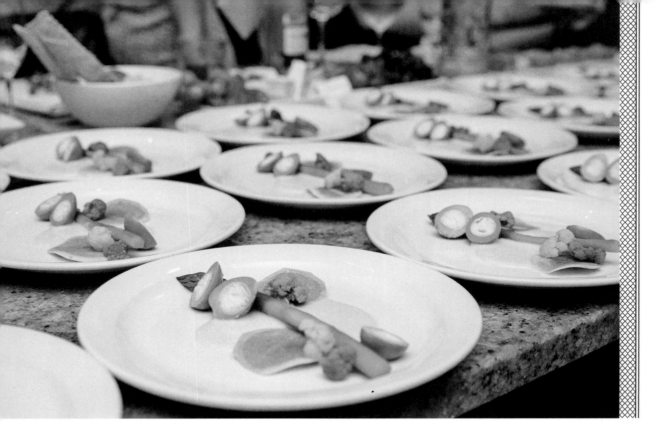

PAIRING CANNABIS WITH FOOD AND WINE

If you've experimented with cannabis, you might have noticed that different strains share similar aromas and flavors with the ingredients that you cook with or the wine that's in your glass. Similar to grape varieties, each strain is unique in its own way, showcasing varying looks, smells, tastes, and effects, which are all greatly influenced by terpenes.

If you tap into your senses, you can learn to recognize the differences between each terpene and apply this knowledge to craft cannabis, food, and wine pairings at home. In other words, think of your hemp as a sommelier would think about a wine. By comparing or contrasting cannabis terpene aroma and flavor profiles with your favorite wines or the ingredients in your cuisine, you can create the perfect pairings.

The most important factor to consider when pairing cannabis, wine, and food is the actual taste of the pairing and matching or contrasting aromas and flavors. My number one recommendation is to get to know your terpene profiles (see the chart opposite). You'll also want to learn how to identify aromas and flavors in your wine and pay close attention to the ingredients that you are cooking with. Evaluate all three side by side during a meal. First, start with the wine (sniff, taste), move on to your cannabis (sniff, taste), and then have a bite of food. Repeat or try this in reverse order to see how the flavors and aromas change.

The goal when creating a pairing is for all of the components to enhance each other. You might even be surprised if the combination creates an entirely new flavor not yet experienced in the food, wine, or cannabis alone. This is what I call "discovering your herbal palate."

While joints are fun to pair with a meal, be aware that the smoke may affect your palate during tastings. For best results, I recommend using a dry flower vaporizer (see Resources on page 206), so you can actually taste the true terpenes alongside your meal without any smoke taint. This will also help keep your pairings balanced so one component doesn't overpower the other.

Chef Holden Jagger, a professional cannabis chef based in Los Angeles, specializes in pairing cannabis with cuisine. As a cultivator, he has a unique relationship to the plant as an ingredient, and as a self-taught "ganjier," he is an expert at matching the flavors in cannabis with the flavors in food. Chef Holden has a gift for finding the perfect combination. Look for one of his favorite pairings on page 172.

Here is my Herb Somm pairing guide that you can reference and use as a cheat sheet. It includes a few CBD-rich cannabis strains for you to experiment with.

	Myrcene	Limonene	Alpha-Pinene	Beta Caryophyllene	Nerolidol	Linalool
Aromas	Earthy Mixed Herbs Mushroom Forest Floor Skunk Mango	Lemon Lime Grapefruit Blood Orange Tangerine	Pine Trees Pine Needle Wet Wood Rosemary Dill	Clove Black Pepper Cinnamon	Perfume Jasmine Ginger Flower Tea Tree	Citrus Blossom Violet Lavender Rose Lilies Geranium
Terpene Benefits	Sleep Aid Muscle Relaxant Anti-depressant	Stress Reliever Weight Loss Aid Mood Enhancer	Aids Asthma Provides Energy Anti-inflammatory	Anti-anxiety Anti-inflammatory Antioxidant Pain Reliever	Antifungal Anti-depressant Sleep Aid	Anti-anxiety Sleep Aid Muscle Relaxant Anti-depressant Anti-acne
Cannabis Strains	Cannatonic Critical Mass Harlequin Harle-Tsu	Lemon Haze OG Kush Tangie	ACDC Jack Herer Trainwreck Valentine X	Omrita RX Northern Lights Skywalker OG Dancehall	Island Sweet Skunk Skywalker OG Banana Kush	Pink Kush Lavender OG LA Confidential Amnesia Haze
Terpene Effect	Sleepy Sedated	Enhanced Mood Uplifted	Alert Focused	Reduced Pain Calm Stress Free	Tranquil Peaceful	Relaxed Rejuvenated
Food Pairings	Mushroom Risotto Spinach Quiche Truffle Popcorn	Oysters Seared Scallops Lemon Bar	Pesto Pasta Sautéed Pine Nuts Rosemary Popcorn	Seared Spiced Steak Chipotle Spiced Nuts Pumpkin Pie	Coconut Jasmine Rice Ginger Honey Chicken Carrot Ginger Cake	Vegan Curry Herbes de Provence Créme Brûlée Honey
Wine Pairings	Pinot Noir Syrah Grenache	Chardonnay Sauvignon Blanc Albariño	Pinot Gris Vermentino New Zealand Sauvignon Blanc	Zinfandel Carbernet Sauvignon Petit Sirah	Rosé Torrontés Gewürztraminer	Muscat Riesling Viognier Nebbiolo

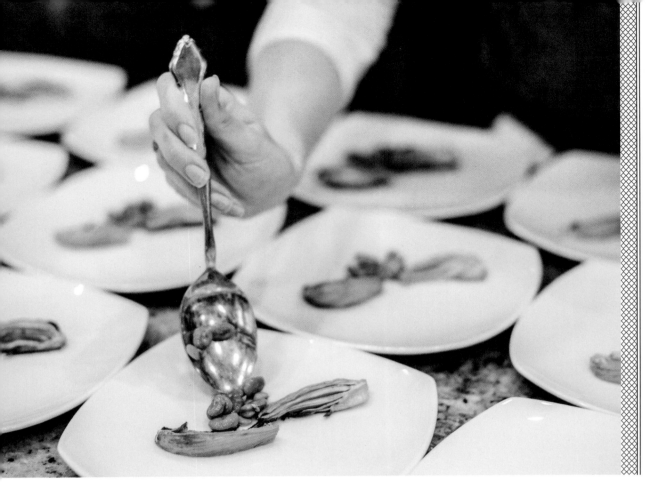

When serving others, plating allows you to customize each guest's dose based on their preference. Using a teaspoon or measured eyedropper will allow you to precisely microdose small bites and appetizers during an infused feast.

TIPS & TRICKS FOR CREATING INFUSED CUISINE

Now that you know the infused food basics, there are a few additional tips and tricks that you'll want to take into consideration before jumping in and making your own recipes. The following tools and suggestions are meant to help you as you begin this culinary journey.

FROM THE CHEF'S KITCHEN

As you begin to cook with cannabis, you'll want to source fresh, wholesome ingredients that highlight the unique characteristics of the dish you're preparing. One of the most important ingredients to source is the actual cannabis or hemp that you'll be incorporating into the recipe. If you are planning to use professionally made hemp CBD oil or a CBD isolate powder, do your research before adding it to your food. Know where your product comes from and how it's made.

Also, keep in mind that many premade CBD oils have added flavors such as peppermint, lavender, etc. While some of these flavors can work in certain recipes (i.e., beverage recipes), I wouldn't advise using them in your food because the essential oils and flavor extracts can easily overpower other ingredients. Instead, source an unflavored full-spectrum CBD oil that's been made with olive oil.

Remember, cannabis buds, leaves, and stems, all contain different aromas, flavors, and varying levels of cannabinoids. Chef Corren Carroll believes the entire plant is fit for consumption. She loves cooking with bold flavors and ingredients. Chocolate is a great example, as it complements and smooths the flavor of the cannabis.

Chef Holden Jagger finds the natural "funky flavors" to be the most exciting part of incorporating herbal products into the dining experience, while Monica Lo and Chef Calvin Eng love to use international flavors highlighting unique ingredients from their background such as fermented bean curd, chile peppers, yuzu, and fish sauce.

As you can see, there are many ingredients that work well with cannabis and hemp. Keep these in mind as you practice the art of pairing with different terpene profiles.

DOSING

You can approach infused foods as you would infused drinks. Start on the low side of the dosage range and adjust upward until you find a perfect balance that works for you. Here are some other recommendations on how to find your ideal dose when mixing CBD (and THC) into food.

Depending on what products you use in a recipe, dosages will vary. For beginners, a good place to start is between 15 to 30 milligrams of CBD and 1 to 5 milligrams of THC per serving, and then adjust accordingly. Remember, you can't have too much of CBD, but the opposite is true for THC. If you're using a cannabis product that contains both, be sure to factor in both cannabinoids as you adjust dosages up or down based on your needs.

If you need to increase the dosage per serving in a recipe, feel free to do so. Just make sure the ingredient ratios that are listed remain the same, so the recipe turns out the way it's supposed to. For instance, you wouldn't want to add more CBD oil than what your recipe calls for to increase the milligrams. Instead, use a different product that contains a higher potency per serving in your recipe.

Lighter, easily digestible infused foods are known to set in faster than dense, rich recipes. When they finally do kick in, CBD effects will be very subtle (i.e., you're not going to feel high or stoned), but THC effects should offer some enhanced euphoric effects. You'll know when THC hits you.

READY-TO-USE GOURMET CBD PRODUCTS

If you're in a rush, sometimes it's easier to use a professionally made product to infuse a recipe. I am a big fan of using premade infused CBD olive oils, honey, ghee, and cooking powder, which can be found online or at a licensed dispensary. You can think of these items as gourmet CBD products. For a full listing of my favorite brands, see Resources on page 206.

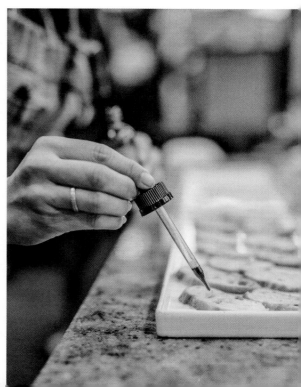

EVERYTHING YOU NEED TO KNOW
ABOUT CBD OLIVE OIL

featuring Yannick Crespo, founder & producer of Pot d'Huile Gourmet Infused Olive Oil

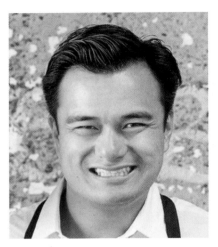

Born in California and raised in the Philippines, Yannick Crespo is a CBD olive oil expert and founder of the gourmet infused olive oil company, Pot d'Huile. Pot d'Huile's line of cannabis- and hemp-infused olive oil products are the premier solution for both culinary professionals and home cooks. Based in San Francisco, Pot d'Huile pairs the highest quality cannabis flower with certified extra-virgin olive oil, sourced from family farms in Northern California. Follow Yannick @potdhuile.

Yannick Crespo: "CBD olive oil is truly a superfood! Not only does it contain CBD, but it also contains polyphenols, which are the medicinal components of olive oil that contain and deliver a wealth of micronutrients and antioxidants to the body—which is similar to what we're discovering about cannabinoids.

When picking out a CBD olive oil, go for the full-spectrum options. Full-spectrum CBD olive oil—as with all full-spectrum CBD products—is generally more effective because of the entourage effect between all the associated cannabinoids and terpenes. Also, look at the packaging—the more helpful the information is on the label, the better the product. A high-quality CBD olive oil should have a 'made on' date, as well as a 'use by' date listed.

All good olive oils have a shelf life of 2 years when stored properly, CBD olive oil included. Good CBD olive oil should also have test results that the producer can provide upon request. It's great to know where and when the CBD olive oil was processed plus the details about the base oil and its certifications. Is it first cold pressed or cold extracted? Is it organic? Is it Non-GMO Project verified? What kind of olive varietals are used and what are their flavor profiles? Where were the olives harvested? All this information indicates that whoever is producing the product truly cares about quality, giving the consumer transparency into the product they are buying.

Once you find a reliable product and are ready to start cooking, remember, the boiling point for CBD and polyphenols hovers around 320°F to 356°F (160°C to 180°C). Knowing this, it's best to use over low heat or simply drizzle it on top of your favorite foods. One of my favorite ways to enjoy CBD olive oil is with a hunk of good, crusty bread!

Dosing is different for everyone. If you're hosting an infused dinner, I recommend infusing sauces and letting a guest dial their own dose. Sauces and dressings are a great way to provide different kinds of flavor options. Include a dropper or a measuring spoon for accurate dosing. If you'd rather infuse the food on your own before serving, that's fine, too. Just clearly mark the dose in each course. Go low and slow, particularly with THC olive oil. As they say, 'You can always have more, but you can't have less.' Feel free to be more liberal with CBD olive oil. Good luck and enjoy!"

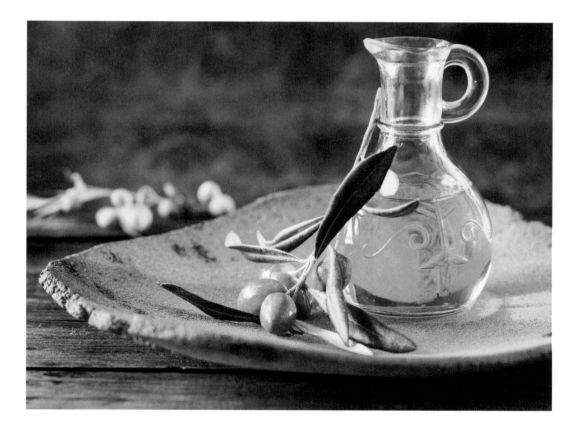

MISTAKES TO AVOID

Over the years, I've made plenty of mistakes when it comes to preparing meals at home. Creating infused foods presents even more obstacles, but you can easily overcome them with a little bit of practice and knowledge. As you've learned, forgetting to decarboxylate your cannabis is a common mistake. Here are a few others to avoid when creating infused foods.

Mistake #1: Overheating Your Cannabinoids & Terpenes

Volatile cannabinoids and terpenes do not like high heat. A common mistake that beginners often make is overheating your infusions or decarboxylating at the wrong temperatures, which degrades the precious compounds that you are trying to preserve. See page 54 for my activation and boiling point guide as you begin to cook.

Mistake #2: Dosing Too High for THC (or Too Low for CBD)

Learning how to estimate dosing is not an easy task. If you are making an infusion using cannabis or hemp flower, you'll have to do some math to estimate the final cannabinoid percentages per serving. This is especially important if you are making THC-infused foods. Depending on what materials and method you use for the infusion, you could end up with a super potent butter or oil that would rock even the most experienced cannabis user. This can happen if you don't use a scale to measure everything properly.

Before adding an infused oil or butter to a recipe, also make sure to try it on its own to gauge how precise your calculation estimates are. Sample ¼ teaspoon and see how you feel. This should help you determine what an appropriate dosage should be per serving. Also be aware that cannabinoids will cook off when baked, roasted, etc., therefore it's important to calculate loss. A rule of thumb that Chef Coreen Carroll goes by is a 13 percent loss of THC or CBD will occur if you bake your edibles at 350°F (177°C) for 30 minutes.

If you are using pure CBD to infuse your recipes, a common mistake is dosing too low. When using an isolated product, you are already missing out on other beneficial terpenes and cannabinoids; to receive the best results, ideally, you should dose higher than you would with other forms of products.

Mistake #3: Not Being Patient after Eating an Edible

Patience is key to any edible or infused cuisine experience. After you consume a food item that contains CBD or THC, be aware it might take up to 2 hours for effects to kick in. Remember, eating CBD-infused foods in higher doses can't impair you. On the other hand, don't get antsy and eat more THC-infused food if you don't feel anything right away.

Pro Tip

As you know, there are many methods to creating an infusion. The method that I prefer for CBD-rich flower involves adding water to butter and coconut oil infusions (or other materials that solidify in the refrigerator) when creating these infusions at home. I prefer this method because it helps clarify and purify your end results by helping remove strong herbal flavors and green notes. Some chefs call this step the "water purge" as you are purging out unattractive characteristics that can affect the flavor and appearance of your recipes.

Chef Coreen Carroll also prefers to use water in her infusions because water helps regulate temperatures and protects the oil and butter from scorching, which in turn will make your infusion taste bitter. Adding water to your infusion will not decrease the potency of your end results. CBD and THC do not bind to water, so be sure your recipe contains enough fat for these precious cannabinoids and other compounds to bind to.

SERVING TIPS

Much like serving infused beverages, if you are entertaining with infused foods, be sure to label everything clearly and precisely. If you are also serving non-infused foods (which you should have available), keep them separate from the elevated cuisine so there is a clear distinction of what is what. At some of the events that I've hosted, I've set up a non-infused food display for people to snack on and then offered tray-passed CBD or THC appetizers for guests to experiment with. Tray passing is a good option, because your server can tell your guests that the food is infused and relay how many milligrams are in each serving.

For formal dining experiences, if you are planning on incorporating THC, it's best to start with low-dose infused appetizers and then showcase the nonintoxicating compounds of cannabis, such as CBD throughout the rest of your menu. That way THC effects will kick in early and by the end of the meal, your guests will feel rounded out by the CBD that they've consumed. There is an art to orchestrating the experience.

Looking to serve alcohol with infused cuisine? Remember the golden rule, "start low, go slow." Do not exceed 5 milligrams of THC throughout the entire meal. This is considered a low-dose, which is the key to a successful dining experience. Think of alcohol as an accent piece—it's not meant to impair you.

If you're planning to host a formal infused dining experience, always provide a printed menu that lists how many milligrams of CBD and THC are in each course.

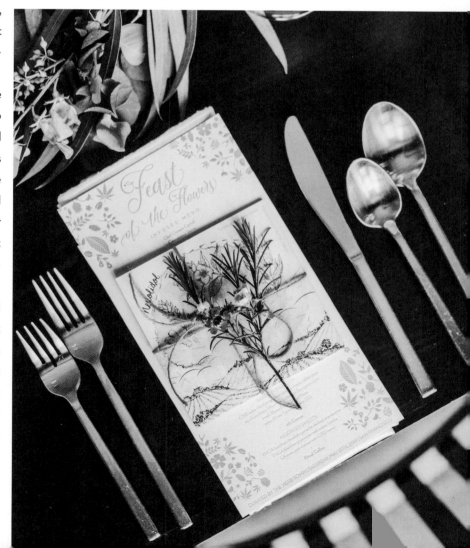

COOKING & ENTERTAINING WITH CBD, THC, AND OTHER COMPONENTS OF CANNABIS

featuring Chef Coreen Carroll, head chef & co-founder of the Cannaisseur Series

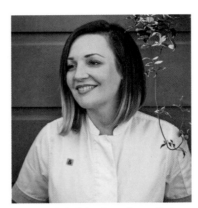

Chef Coreen Carroll is the co-founder and head chef of the Cannaisseur Series, one of San Francisco's most acclaimed pop-up dining events that features seasonal cannabis cuisine expertly paired with artisan flower. Chef Coreen's meals and recipes have enchanted foodies across the nation who wish to elevate fine dining by incorporating cannabis into their cuisine. Chef Coreen collaborated with Chef Stephanie Hua, cannabis pioneer and founder of Mellows, on the 2018 cookbook Edibles: Small Bites for the Modern Cannabis Kitchen *published by Chronicle Books. Follow chef Coreen @frauleinchef and @cannaisseurseries or visit CannaisseurSeries.com*

Chef Coreen Carroll: "In 2015 I founded the Cannaisseur Series with my husband, Ryan Bush. We learned early on that you can't just pump a bunch of THC into a room full of guests for four straight hours or many of them would not make it through the night. Because I am a believer in consuming the full spectrum of the cannabis flower, we decided to take our guests on a curated journey that allows them to learn and taste the different parts of the plant. We generally like to frontload the THC consumption, so guests are really only eating or drinking THC within the first hour or two. Throughout the rest of the event, I pair dishes infused with nonintoxicating components such as canna leaves, terpenes, CBD, THCA, and CBDA alongside intermezzos of THC & CBD flower joints and vapes. We also keep a ton of CBD-infused water on the table throughout the meal, giving guests a way to modulate their high, ensuring everyone stays at a nice even level. Each person has a completely different tolerance level and creating a space that is welcoming to both the novice and the experienced consumer is extremely important to us.

Living in the Bay Area, an epicenter for the cannabis industry, really gives me a vast variety of cannabis components to cook with. I generally make a lot of my own infusions with either flower I grew myself or that was produced by one our cannabis industry friends. For anyone looking to cook at home, you can visit just about any dispensary these days to find a huge variety of products that can be used to make your own in-home infusions. You'll also find already infused products, such as tinctures and olive oils, that can be incorporated into your dishes. To try out cooking with cannabis on your own, I've provided the following recipe for my Cannaisseur Puffs, a fan favorite at most Cannaisseur events. I've also created a delicious recipe for Salmon Gravlax with Cucumber & Zesty CBD Tarragon Dijon (page 178), which I think you'll enjoy!"

CANNAISSEUR PUFFS

YIELD: **24** puffs

TARGET DOSE: 5 mg CBD | 0.33 THC per puff
(using CBD-Rich Flower Butter, page 64) or 5 mg CBD per puff
(using CBD Isolate Butter, page 65)

EQUIPMENT
Baking pan
Medium saucepan
Mixing bowl
Parchment paper or silicone baking
    mat
Wooden flat spatula
Standing kitchen mixer with paddle
    attachment
Piping bag
Whisk

½ cup (79 g) white rice flour
¼ cup (48 g) potato starch
2 tablespoons (19 g) tapioca
⅔ cup (160 ml) water
4 tablespoons (56 g) CBD butter of
    your choice (page 64 and 65)
1½ teaspoons sugar
½ teaspoon kosher salt
3 large eggs
½ packed cup (60 g) shredded
    Emmentaler Alpine Swiss
2 tablespoons (6 g) finely chopped
    fresh canna leaves (optional)

NOTE

*If you're using THC-infused butter and
your canna infusion is too strong, instead of
using 4 tablespoons (56 g) of THC butter,
combine only 1 or 2 tablespoons (14 or 28 g)
with enough regular unsalted butter to equal
4 tablespoons (56 g).*

Preheat the oven to 400°F (200°C). Place the oven rack in the middle. Line a sheet pan with parchment paper or a silicone baking mat. Place the rice flour, potato starch, and tapioca in a medium bowl and whisk until evenly combined.

In a medium saucepan, bring the water, butter, sugar and salt to a boil over medium-high heat. Once it boils, add the flour mixture all at once and stir with a wooden flat spatula. You must work quickly over the heat, stirring carefully at first to avoid spilling. Once the dough comes together and pulls away from the sides of the pan, the stirring will become more difficult. Don't stop and continue to stir until a film begins to form on the bottom of the pan. This will take 1 to 2 minutes.

Immediately remove the saucepan from the heat and pour the batter into a standing kitchen mixer fitted with the paddle attachment. Continue to mix the batter on medium-low speed to allow it to cool down, 3 to 4 minutes.

Once cooled, but still warm, stop the paddle. On medium-high speed, add the eggs one at a time: Allow the mixture to come together after each egg addition. Make sure to scrape the bowl down as well after each addition. It will look like it's separating, but once all of the eggs have been added you should have a smooth and paste-like batter. Add the Emmentaler and canna leaves to the bowl. Allow the mixture to come together once more, making sure to scrape down the sides once or twice.

Add the batter to a piping bag. Cut the tip to make a ¾-inch (2-cm) opening. Pipe twenty-four 1-inch (2.5-cm) mounds, allowing at least 1½ inches (3.5 cm) between each mound. Using wet finger tips, smooth out any points that protrude and gently shape all mounds into circles so they bake and brown evenly. Bake for 25 to 35 minutes until the puffs turn a deep golden brown.

Once done, transfer to a wire rack and allow to cool completely. These are best served immediately. To freeze, store the uncooked batter in an airtight container for up to 3 months. Defrost in refrigerator when ready to use.

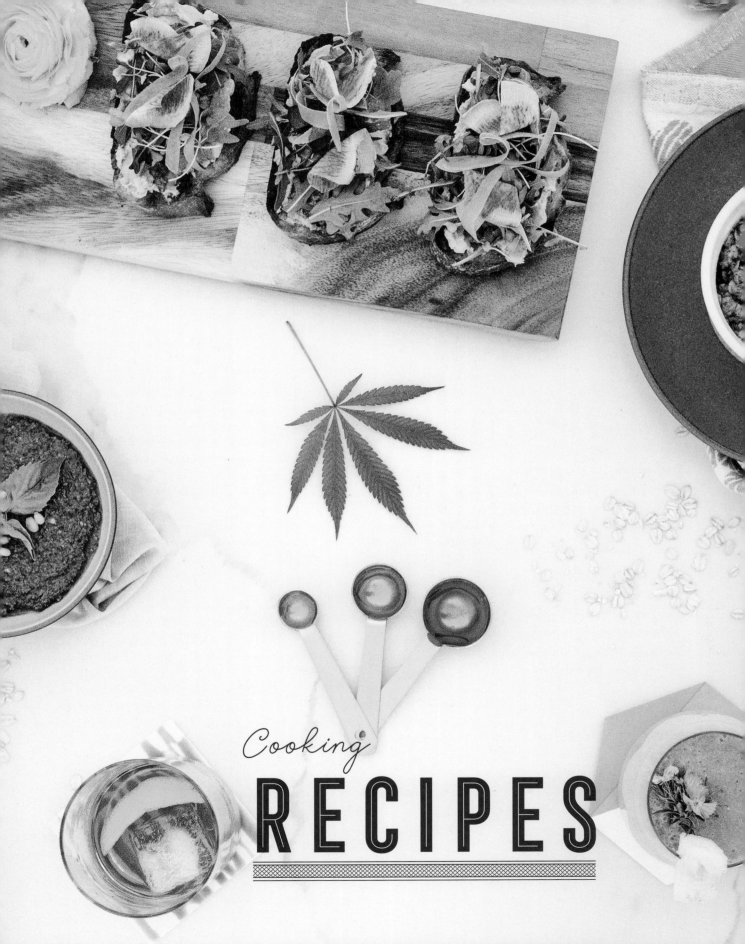

Cooking

RECIPES

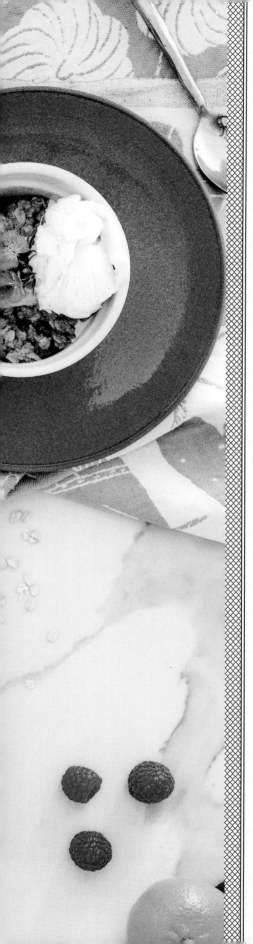

To cook with cannabis properly, you'll need to create CBD olive oil, CBD coconut oil, and CBD butter (see pages 61 and 63 to 65). For these CBD-rich cannabis infusion recipes, I used Harle-Tsu flower that measured at a total of 15 percent CBD and 1 percent THC before decarboxylation. Remember, your numbers will differ depending on the strain and source that you use, so be sure to calculate your own CBD/THC milligrams per serving before making your infusion (see page 52 for at-home dosage calculations). Do your best to make an accurate estimate, and always sample a small portion of each batch before serving to others.

After you create these essential "pantry" ingredients—it's on to the food recipes. If you'd rather take a shortcut and use a commercially made CBD product in your recipes, that's fine, too. There are options for both methods.

The target dose per recipe varies depending on the total servings per item and method used, but note that all of the doses in this chapter fall between 5 and 30 milligrams of CBD per serving, which is considered low on the dosage range. If you prefer a higher dose, use what's best for you and adjust the recipe accordingly. If you're using a premade CBD oil, the dosages indicated in this chapter are based on using a 30-milliliter bottle containing a total of 1,000 milligrams of CBD (or about 33 milligrams CBD per dropper).

Are you ready for the fun part? The infused cuisine included in this chapter is not only delicious but is pleasurable and easy to make. For the more nuanced cannabis enthusiasts, you will also find a collection of more challenging recipes prepared by some of the top cannabis chefs and recipe developers in the cannabis industry. Bon appétit and enjoy responsibly!

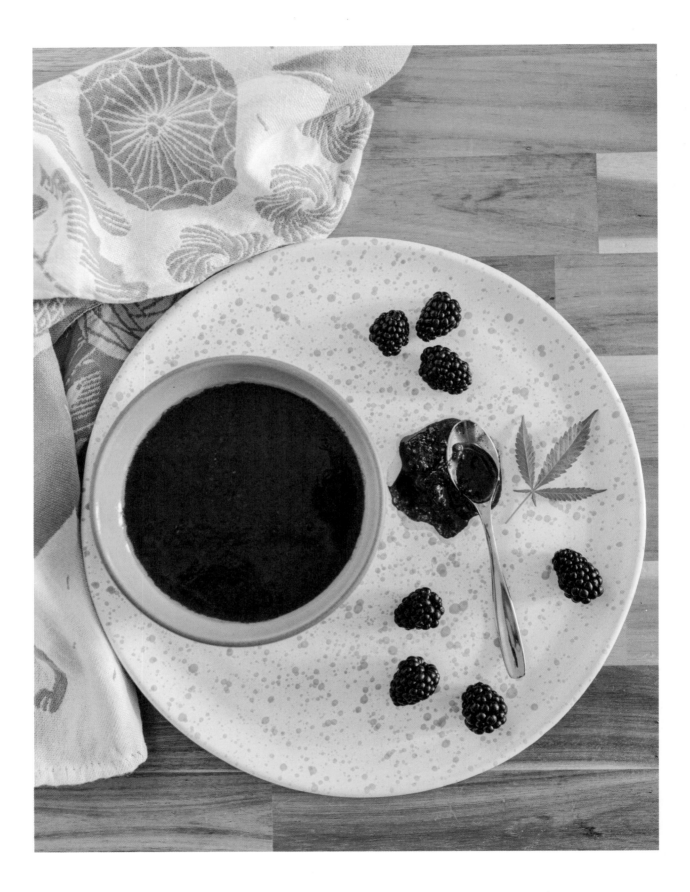

BLACKBERRY BALSAMIC CBD VINAIGRETTE

In the warmer months, I love creating fresh blackberry balsamic CBD vinaigrette, which is the perfect companion to a variety of fresh salads. This CBD-infused vinaigrette takes less than ten minutes to make—a perfect recipe when you're in the mood for something simple yet delicious.

YIELD: ¾ cup (175 ml)	**TARGET DOSE:** 7 mg CBD | 0.50 THC per tablespoon (using CBD Olive Oil, page 61) or about 10 mg CBD per tablespoon (using commercially made CBD oil, see note below)

EQUIPMENT
Measuring cups
Measuring spoons
Small bowl
Small saucepan
One 8-ounce (240-ml) sterilized
     Mason jar

½ cup (70 g) fresh blackberries

¼ cup (60 ml) balsamic vinegar

½ tablespoon (10 g) stone-ground or
     whole-grain mustard

½ tablespoon (8 ml) fresh lemon juice

1 teaspoon honey

3 tablespoons (45 ml) CBD Olive Oil
     (page 61; see note)

3 tablespoons (45 ml) olive oil (add
     more if you prefer a softer taste)

Salt and pepper

In a small sauté pan, heat the blackberries, balsamic vinegar, mustard, lemon juice, and honey. Stir over low heat as the blackberries begin to warm and the honey dissolves. The blackberries should soften in 3 to 4 minutes, but do not let the balsamic boil.

Remove the pan from the heat and transfer the mixture into a small bowl. Using the back of a fork, smash the blackberries into the balsamic mixture until it turns into a soup-like consistency.

Whisk in the CBD olive oil and regular olive oil. Blend until it's mixed together well. Add a dash of salt and pepper to taste. Continue to stir and then transfer to a Mason jar for storage. Let cool before serving and store in the refrigerator to best preserve. Give your new Blackberry Balsamic CBD Vinaigrette a good shake before serving. Eat within 1 to 2 days after making for the freshest flavor.

NOTE

If you don't have time to make your own CBD olive oil, you can still incorporate CBD into this recipe by adding your favorite commercially made CBD oil. Simply mix ¾ teaspoon (123 mg CBD) of unflavored CBD oil of your choice (preferably made with olive oil) with 5 tablespoons plus 2¼ teaspoons (86 ml) of regular olive oil, then follow the directions as written.

CBD PESTO

To liven up a dish, sometimes you need a really great sauce. Look no further than CBD Pesto. Blending together a bounty of fresh and flavorful ingredients, pesto is easy to make and it tastes incredible. I love incorporating feta into this recipe. It adds creaminess and complexity, plus it helps balance out overly pungent garlic flavors. Because CBD oil can often have green notes on the palate, the fresh basil, baby spinach, and Italian parsley perfectly complement the oil's flavors.

YIELD: **16** servings (about 1 cup)	**TARGET DOSE:** 5 mg CBD | 0.375 mg THC per tablespoon (using CBD Olive Oil, page 61) or about 8 mg CBD per tablespoon (using commercially made CBD oil, see note below)

EQUIPMENT
Blender (or food processor)
Measuring cups
Measuring spoons
Small sauté pan

3½ cups (140 g) fresh basil, plus more for garnish

1 cup (30 g) fresh spinach

½ cup (30 g) fresh Italian parsley

½ cup (75 g) cherry tomatoes

2 teaspoons (10 ml) fresh lemon juice

⅓ cup (75 g) feta cheese

3 tablespoons (45 ml) CBD Olive Oil (page 61; see note)

1 tablespoon (9 g) pine nuts, plus 5 or 6 more for garnish

3 large garlic cloves, peeled

Olive oil

Salt and pepper

Place the basil, spinach, and parsley in a blender or food processor along with the tomatoes, lemon juice, feta, and CBD olive oil. Set aside.

In a small sauté pan over medium-low heat, sauté the pine nuts and garlic in a splash of olive oil for about 2 minutes or until the pine nuts turn golden brown. Remove from the heat and add the ingredients to the blender or food processor. Add a dash of salt and pepper. Blend until the mixture is finely chopped and pesto becomes a smooth, thick sauce.

Using a spoon, scoop the pesto sauce into a small bowl and top with an airtight lid. Garnish with pine nuts, basil, and a dash of olive oil.

NOTE *If you don't have time to make your own CBD olive oil, you can still incorporate CBD into this recipe by adding your favorite commercially made CBD oil. Simply mix ¾ teaspoon (123 mg CBD) of unflavored CBD oil of your choice (preferably made with olive oil) with 2 tablespoons plus 2¼ teaspoons (41 ml) of regular olive oil, then follow the directions as noted.*

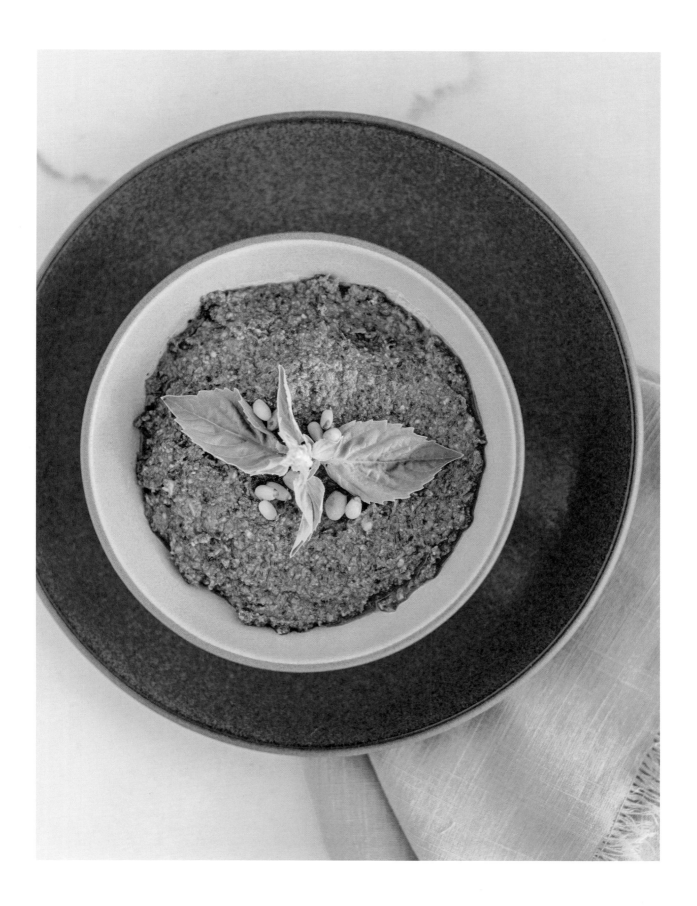

PREPARING VEGAN CUISINE & EXPLORING CANNABIS PAIRINGS

featuring Chef Holden Jagger, head chef & co-founder of Altered Plates

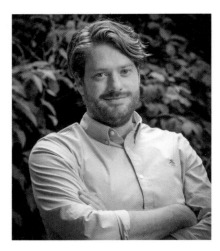

Chef Holden Jagger has a long, passionate relationship with both cooking and cannabis. As a chef who cultivates, Holden also has access to the cannabis plant at many stages of its growth and truly believes in looking at cannabis as a vegetable and exploring inventive uses for the nonintoxicating parts of the plant. Chef Holden was listed on Green State's Top Ten Cannabis Chefs in the Country in 2017 and was a Zagat 30 Under 30 recipient. In 2016, Chef Holden and his sister, Rachel Burkons, founded Altered Plates, a Los Angeles-based creative culinary collective that brings together cannabis, food, beverage, and good old-fashioned hospitality. Altered Plates was the first culinary team to host a terpene-inspired dinner at the James Beard House in New York City in 2019. Follow Chef Holden Jagger @ChefHoldenJagger.

Chef Holden Jagger: "Cooking vegan dishes is a nice challenge for chefs trained in classic French techniques. As a young cook, I watched 55-pound (25 kg) blocks of butter disappear in a night—I was always concerned with the impact of that. A plant-based lifestyle is not a personal choice of mine, but it is a lifestyle that I support as a chef. For those who eat vegan and plant-based diets, I believe that they deserve creative, delicious food, full of texture, flavor, and depth. As a chef it is my job to serve my guests something they want to eat, while still being something that I want to cook. Knowing this, I've created a fun and flavorful vegan recipe for Carrots al Pastor with charred avocado, cashew lime cream, and puffed amaranth. If you're looking to pair cannabis with this dish via smoking or vaping (refer back to pages 27 and 157), the spices in my recipe will pair perfectly with a high alpha-Pinene CBD-rich varietal like ACDC. The rich smoke will offset some of the heat, and the herbaceous notes will fill some space between the creamy avocado. I highly recommend trying out this pairing to explore a new world of flavors and aromas that are created when you combine cannabis with food. This is a different take on how you can incorporate CBD flower into the dining experience."

CARROTS AL PASTOR *with* CHARRED AVOCADO, CASHEW LIME CREAM, *and* PUFFED AMARANTH

Recipe by Chef Holden Jagger, Altered Plates

YIELD: 6 servings	CBD Flower Pairing: ACDC

EQUIPMENT
Baking tray
Blender
Cast iron skillet
Medium saucepan
Sauté pan
Squeeze bottle

CASHEW LIME CREAM
½ cup (70 g) raw cashews

6 tablespoons (90 ml) water, plus more as needed

Zest and juice of 1 lime

½ teaspoon white vinegar

1 teaspoon salt

1 tablespoon (5 g) nutritional yeast

CHARRED AVOCADO
2 tablespoons (40 g) avocado honey

1 tablespoon (15 ml) avocado oil

¼ teaspoon salt

Pepper

2 ripe avocados

1 to 2 tablespoons (15 to 30 ml) olive oil

PUFFED AMARANTH
¼ cup (52 g) white amaranth

To make the cashew lime cream: Boil 1½ (355 ml) cups of water. Pour the boiling water over the raw cashews, and set aside for 10 minutes. Drain and place the cashews into a blender with the 6 tablespoons (90 ml) of water, lime zest, lime juice, vinegar, salt, and nutritional yeast. Blend until a smooth paste forms, adding additional water if needed to get the right consistency. Storing this in a squeeze bottle will help when plating.

To make the charred avocado: In a small bowl, combine the honey, avocado oil, salt, and pepper. Heat a sauté pan over medium heat. Halve and pit the avocados and using a pastry brush, glaze the avocados with the honey mixture, leaving the skin on. Add oil to the warm pan and place the glazed avocados in the pan flesh-side down. Cook until they are golden brown and deeply caramelized. Season and set aside until ready to plate.

To make the amaranth: Heat a large saucepot over medium heat and when smoking hot add the amaranth 1 tablespoon (13 g) at a time. The amaranth will pop wildly like popcorn. Swirl the pot over the flame and pour out the puffed amaranth onto a sheet tray before it scorches. Repeat until all the amaranth is puffed.

Preheat the oven to 350°F (177°C).

(continued)

CARROTS AL PASTOR

2 dried guajillo chiles

½ cup (120 ml) pineapple juice

Juice of 1 lime

2 cloves garlic, peeled

¼ white onion

1 teaspoon salt

½ teaspoon dried oregano

Pinch ground cinnamon

1 ounce (28 g) achiote paste

1 pound colored carrots (about 2 small bunches), washed, tops trimmed, and split lengthwise

To make the carrots al pastor: In a cast iron skillet on medium-low heat, toast the guajillo chilies for about 3 minutes or until fragrant. Remove from the heat and clean the peppers of their stems and seeds. Take care, wear latex gloves, and avoid touching your face. Also take time to remove the veins of the peppers where the heat is concentrated. Take the clean peppers and submerge them in a bowl of ice water for 30 minutes.

Add the drained guajillo chiles, pineapple juice, lime juice, garlic, onion, salt, oregano, cinnamon, and achiote paste to a blender. Blend until very smooth, about 1 minute.

Reserve a ½ cup (120 ml) of the sauce. Place the prepared carrots in a large bowl and, wearing gloves, liberally coat the carrots with the rest of the sauce. Lay the coated carrots on a sheet tray and roast them in the oven for 30 to 35 minutes, until tender and well roasted.

To plate: Scoop a one-quarter of the charred avocado onto the plate making room for the carrots. Place the carrots over the avocado. Top with the cashew cream and liberally coat with puffed amaranth.

To pair: I recommend pairing this dish with CBD-rich ACDC. Try taking a puff of smoke in your mouth before tasting a dish, or try the ACDC after you take a bite. You'll notice there is a beautiful synergy of flavors on the palate.

AVOCADO CBD SPRING TOAST

During the spring and summer months, the best avocado, vegetables, and fresh herbs are in abundance, which means they could be a perfect match for your next avocado toast creation. This recipe can be enjoyed any time of day, but it especially makes an excellent appetizer for your friends. For some extra flavor, add a dollop of CBD Pesto (page 170) on the side to dip the toast into. Trust me, it's scrumptious.

YIELD: **4** servings	**TARGET DOSE:** 14 mg CBD ǀ 1 mg THC per toast (using CBD Olive Oil, page 61) or 17 mg CBD per toast (using commercially made CBD oil, see note below)

TOAST

4 thick slices of freshly baked bread or bread of your choice

Extra-virgin olive oil

Salt (optional)

AVOCADO SPREAD

1½ avocados, peeled and pitted

1 tablespoon (15 ml) fresh lemon juice

2 tablespoons (30 ml) CBD Olive Oil (page 61; see note)

1 teaspoon red pepper flakes (reduce to ½ teaspoon if you're sensitive to heat)

Salt and pepper

TOPPINGS

1 cup (30 g) arugula or watercress

1 cup (34 g) microgreens

3 baby rainbow carrots, shaved (1 of each color)

1 watermelon radish, shaved (use best looking pieces to top toast with)

Salt and pepper

2 tablespoons (30 ml) CBD Olive Oil (page 61)

SIDES (optional, but highly recommended)

CBD Pesto (page 170)

EQUIPMENT

Small sauté pan or griddle

Basting brush

Spatula

Potato masher

Small mixing bowl

To make the toast: Heat a sauté pan or griddle over medium heat. Using a basting brush, coat both sides of the bread slices with olive oil to taste. Toast the bread, flipping it consistently using a spatula, and cook until it's crispy on both sides. Sprinkle with salt (if using) and set aside.

To make the avocado spread: Place the avocados into a small mixing bowl and mash them using a potato masher. Add the lemon juice, CBD oil, red pepper flakes, salt, and pepper. Stir until blended well.

To serve: Spread the CBD avocado mixture on top of the toast. Top evenly with arugula, microgreens, rainbow carrots, and watermelon radish. Add a dash of salt and pepper, and drizzle with the CBD olive oil evenly on top to taste. For an extra delicious touch, serve with a side of CBD pesto for dipping.

NOTE

If you don't have time to make your own CBD olive oil, you can still incorporate CBD into this recipe by adding your favorite commercially made CBD oil. Simply mix 2 droppers full (66 mg CBD) of unflavored CBD oil of your choice (preferably made with olive oil) with 1 tablespoon plus 2½ teaspoons (26 ml) extra-virgin olive oil, then add to the avocado spread as directed.

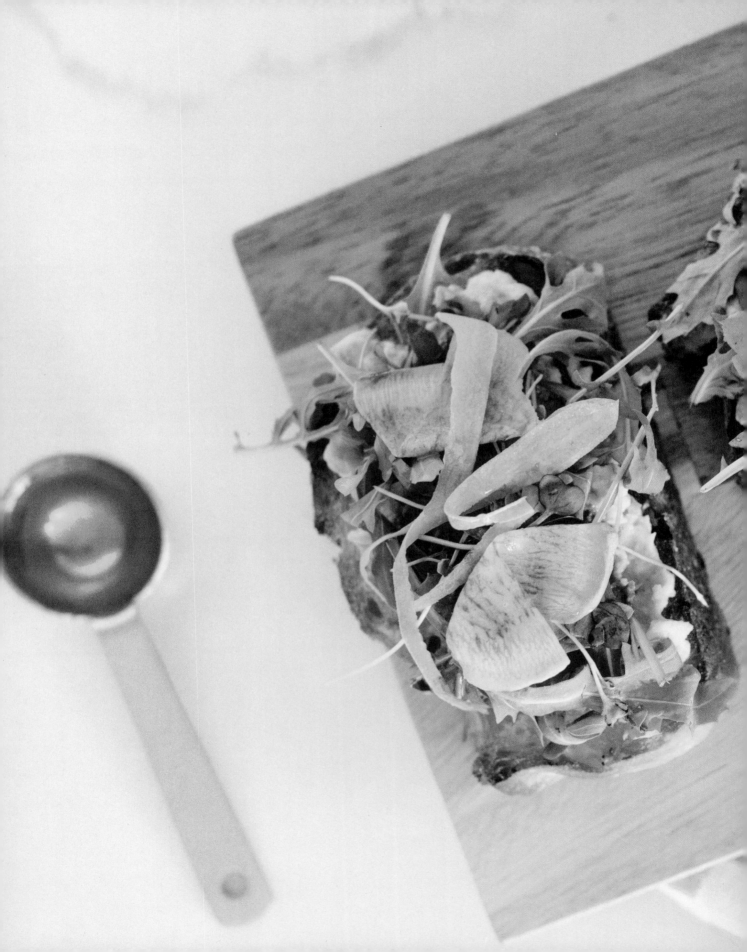

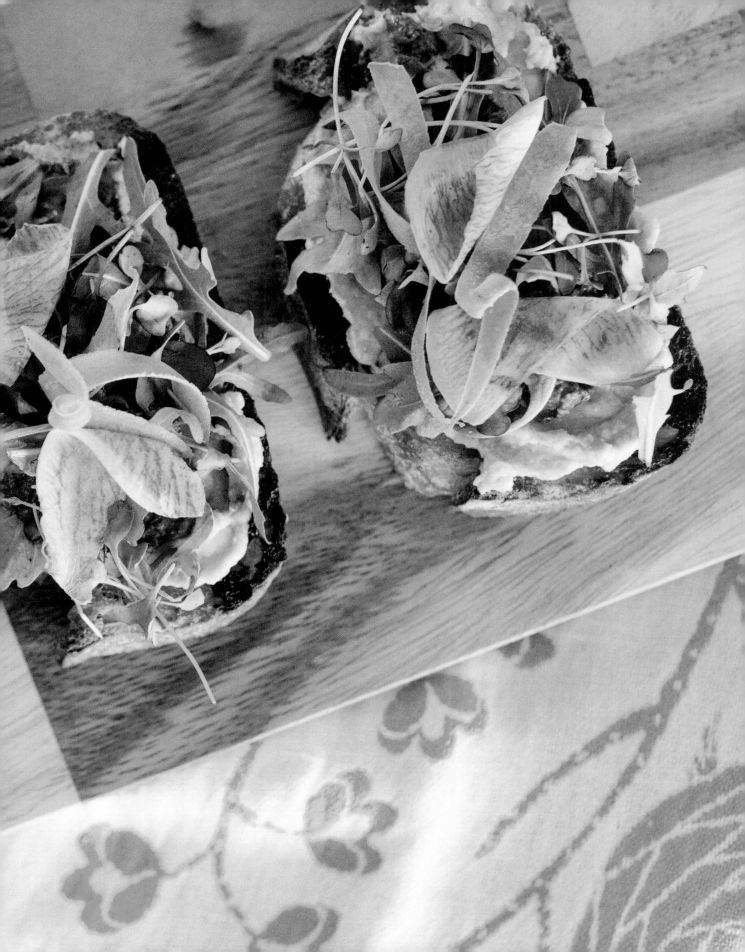

SALMON GRAVLAX *with* CUCUMBER & ZESTY CBD TARRAGON DIJON

Recipe by Chef Coreen Carroll, Cannaisseur Series

Known as one of the ultimate easy-to-make luxury foods, salmon gravlax is not only delicious, but it's beautiful to look at when plated. Chef Corren Carroll's recipe is perfect for serving as an appetizer or tapa dish. Combining the delicious flavors of freshly cured salmon, cucumber, and zesty CBD tarragon Dijon, this twist on the classic Nordic dish will become a quick favorite in your home.

YIELD: **10** servings	**TARGET DOSE:** 6 mg CBD | 0.4 mg THC per serving (using CBD Olive Oil, page 61) or 8 mg CBD per serving (using commercially made CBD oil, see note below)

EQUIPMENT

Mixing bowl
Plastic wrap
Sharp fillet knife
Canned goods or oil tins (something weighing at least 5 pounds [2.3 kg])

---

3 to 4½ pounds (1.4 to 2 kg) skin-on salmon fillet, cleaned and deboned

1 cup (48 g) chopped fresh cannabis leaves or **(16 g) fresh cilantro**

½ cup (32 g) chopped fresh dill

2 tablespoons (10 g) whole coriander, crushed

1½ cups (300 g) sugar

1 cup (150 g) kosher salt

¼ cup (32 g) whole white peppercorns, cracked

¼ cup (24 g) whole allspice, cracked

1 pound (454 g) cucumber, mixed varietals (Parisian, Japanese, English, Lemon, etc.)

Prepare the salmon by removing any pin bones or unwanted fatty edges. Do not remove the skin. Cut the salmon down its center into 2 equal-size pieces that can evenly line up when laid on top of each other. Combine the herbs and crushed coriander in a bowl and set aside. Mix the sugar, salt, pepper, and allspice in a medium bowl until well combined.

Spread 1 cup of the salt mixture into the bottom of a small flat dish large enough to hold your salmon fillets. Lay one fillet of fish on the salt, skin-side down. Sprinkle ½ cup (75 g) of the salt mixture over the flesh side, covering the top and edges of the one fish fillet. Scatter all of the chopped herbs and coriander on top of the salted fish fillet. Add an additional ½ cup (75 g) of the salt mixture over the herbs, making sure everything stays on top of the fillet. Place the second half of the salmon on top, skin-side up. Sprinkle with the remaining salt mixture on top, making sure to cover the sides. Wash your hands and wrap the entire dish in plastic wrap until fully covered and enclosed. The tighter the better.

Cover the wrapped fish with another plate or small pan. Place it in the refrigerator. Weigh the plate down with something weighing at least 5 pounds (2.3 kg). The idea is for the fish to cure and juices to extract; adding some pressure helps this process.

Refrigerate for 2 to 4 days total, depending on the size of the fish. Make sure to turn your fish halfway through curing (bottom to the top, flipped) about 1 to 2 days in, rewrapping again and weighing it down afterward. When cured you will have a rich-colored fish that is slightly firm to the touch. Once cured, remove all salt by washing under cold water. Pat dry very well, and store the fish in an airtight container up to 1 week.

DIJON SAUCE

½ cup (120 g) good-quality Dijon mustard

2 tablespoons (8 g) tarragon, chopped

2 tablespoons (30 ml) CBD Olive Oil (page 61; see note)

1 tablespoon (15 ml) fresh lemon juice

On the day you are serving the fish, make the Dijon sauce: Mix the Dijon, tarragon, CBD olive oil, and lemon juice in a small bowl until well combined. Store in the refrigerator for up to 3 days.

When ready to serve the fish, slice thin ¼-inch (6-mm)-thick slices from the fillet by gliding your dimpled carving knife across the fish. Start on the thick end of the fillet and slice off one piece at a time. Do not slice into the skin. Keep the sliced fish chilled and covered until ready to serve.

The gravlax can be eaten with Dijon sauce alone, or serve it on toast if you would like the dish to be more filling and served as a first or second course. Add sliced and chopped seasonal cucumbers from your area along with the slices of fish and the Dijon.

NOTE

If you don't have time to make your own CBD olive oil, you can still incorporate CBD into this recipe by adding your favorite premade CBD oil. Simply mix ½ teaspoon (82 mg CBD) of unflavored CBD oil of your choice (preferably made with olive oil) with 1 tablespoon plus 2½ teaspoons (26 ml) extra-virgin olive oil, then add to the Dijon as directed.

179

CBD & COOKING

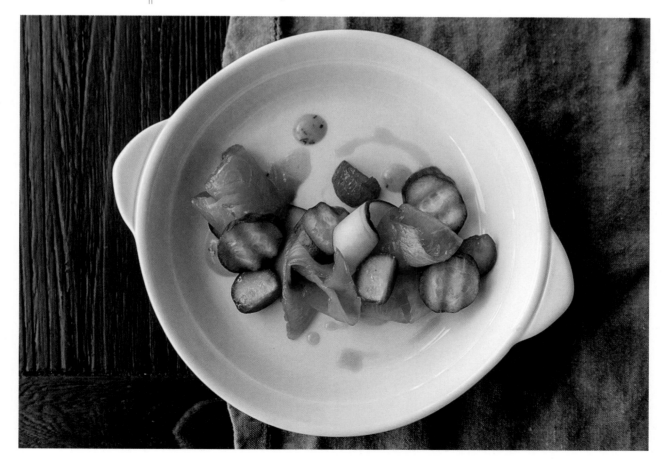

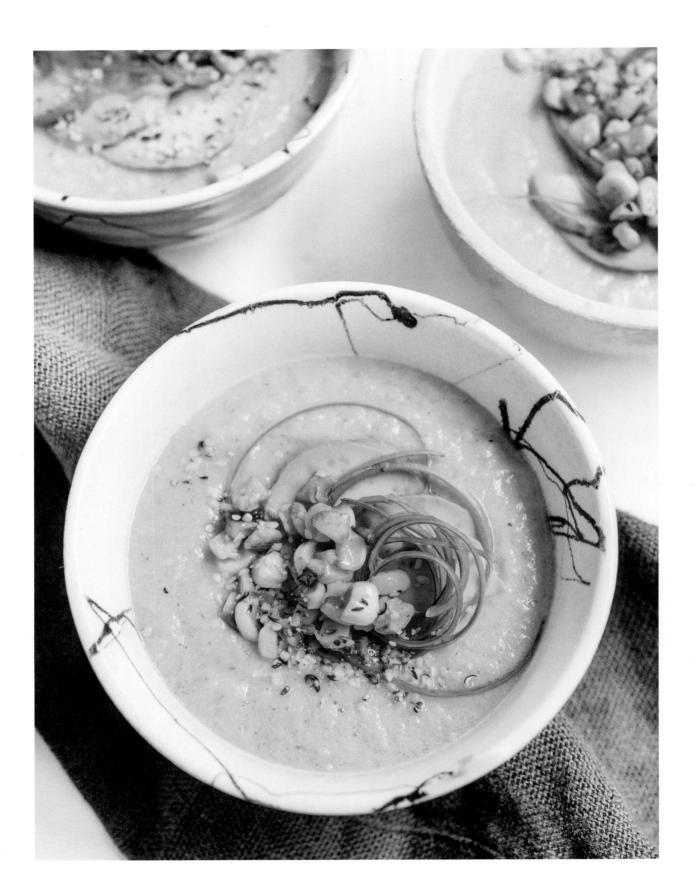

CREAMY *(no cream!)* CBD SWEET CORN CHOWDER

Recipe by Monica Lo, Sous Weed

Every year, as warmer weather approaches and spring arrives sweet corn season begins and it is something to celebrate. To make the most of this flavorful time of year, Monica Lo has developed an out-of-this world delicious dairy-free sweet corn chowder recipe that blends together all the right ingredients. This recipe is quick and easy, taking less than thirty minutes to assemble, which makes it a perfect starter to serve at your next CBD feast.

YIELD: 3 servings	**TARGET DOSE:** your desired dose

EQUIPMENT
Large saucepan
Measuring cups
Measuring spoons
Blender
Small skillet

¼ cup (60 ml) extra-virgin olive oil

1 large shallot, roughly chopped

2 garlic cloves, minced

Kernels from 2 ears sweet corn

4 cups (960 ml) chicken broth

1 ripe avocado, peeled and pitted

Salt and pepper

CHARRED CORN

1 tablespoon (15 ml) extra-virgin olive oil

Kernels from 1 ear sweet corn

2 teaspoons Sous Weed Avocado Oil (page 155; or CBD hemp oil tincture)

Salt

GARNISH

Avocado slices (optional)

1 tablespoon (7 g) hemp hearts

1 scallion, thinly sliced

1 fresh jalapeño pepper, seeds removed, finely diced (optional)

In a large saucepan over medium heat, combine the olive oil, shallot, and garlic. Cook for about 5 minutes, stirring often, until the shallot is translucent. Add the corn kernels and chicken broth, and bring to a simmer. Cook for 10 minutes.

Pour the soup into a blender and add an avocado. When the soup is cool enough to blend, carefully purée on high speed until the soup is creamy. Alternatively, use an immersion blender and blend the soup in the pot. Add salt and pepper, to taste. Pour the soup back into the pot, and reheat it on low while you prepare the charred corn garnish.

To make the charred corn: In a small skillet over medium heat, combine the olive oil and the corn kernels. Let the corn char on the skillet for 4 minutes before stirring. Let the kernels get golden brown for another 3 minutes before removing from the heat. Transfer the corn to a small bowl and pour the Sous Weed avocado oil on top. Add a pinch of salt and mix well.

To serve, ladle the soup into bowls. Garnish with charred corn, avocado (if using), hemp hearts, scallions, and jalapeño (if using).

MASTERING INFUSED RECIPES WITH INTERNATIONAL FLAVORS

featuring Chef Calvin Eng, Professional Chef

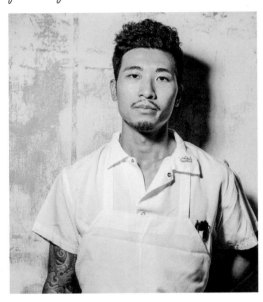

Born and raised in Brooklyn, New York, Chef Calvin Eng comes from a long history of creating delicious international flavors with a focus on highlighting traditional Chinese ingredients. His career as a chef began after studying culinary arts at Johnson & Wales University in Providence, Rhode Island, followed by a number of successful positions in top kitchens including New York City's oldest dim sum establishment, Nom Wah. Currently, he is the Chef de Cuisine at Win Son, one of Brooklyn's hottest Taiwanese-American restaurants. Chef Calvin is also in the R&D phase of making his own line of cannabis-infused Chinese condiments. Follow Chef Calvin @calvinhungry.

Chef Calvin Eng: "Growing up in a Chinese household, I was exposed to funky flavors like fermented bean curd and shrimp paste from a young age. As I delve deeper into Cantonese cuisine, I'm starting to introduce the flavors and ingredients of my childhood into my professional cooking. Chinese cuisine has many dishes that feature oil-based sauces: I've found it quite easy to work cannabis-infused oils into the dishes I grew up eating. The combinations work well together and feel natural. In addition to my professional work as a chef, I also make an infused chili oil that can be used as a condiment on dumplings, a marinade for proteins, a base for different sauces, and even a topping on ice cream. Celebrating international flavors, here is one of my favorite recipes for Fermented Black Beans & Clams."

FERMENTED BLACK BEANS & CLAMS

YIELD: 18 clams

TARGET DOSE: 29 mg CBD | 2 mg THC per clam (using CBD-Rich Flower Butter, page 64) or 30 mg CBD per clam (using CBD Isolate Butter, page 65)

EQUIPMENT

Wok or large pan
Cheesecloth
Sous vide precision cooker
Large pot
Vacuum seal
Vacuum seal bag

18 clams (2½ to 3 pounds, or 1.1 to 1.4 kg) Manila or littleneck clams

1 tablespoon (15 ml) oyster sauce

1 tablespoon (8 g) cornstarch

2 tablespoons (30 ml) water

2 tablespoons (30 ml) canola oil

2 teaspoons (4 g) minced peeled, fresh ginger

2 garlic cloves, minced

2 tablespoons (16 g) fermented black beans

½ or 1 red bird's eye chile pepper, sliced thin (based on your preference)

1 scallion, sliced thin

4 ounces (118 ml) Shaoxing rice wine

4 ounces (118 ml) chicken stock

CBD butter of your choice (pages 64 and 65)

Fresh cilantro, for garnish

1 cup (158 g) cooked white rice

Purge and clean the clams very well in cold water.

Make a slurry with the oyster sauce, cornstarch, and water. Add the canola oil to a wok or pan. When the oil is hot, add the ginger and garlic, and sweat until fragrant. Be careful not to burn, and adjust the heat if needed. Add the fermented black beans, chile pepper, and scallion, and toss to combine. Add the clams and toss gently. Pour in the wine and chicken stock, and steam the clams open with the lid on.

Once the clams are starting to open, pour in the oyster sauce slurry around the edges of wok. Stir and boil until the slurry is incorporated and the sauce has a nice consistency. Taste and adjust the seasoning (oyster sauce, etc.), based on preference.

Cut the heat and emulsify in a desired amount of infused CBD butter. For this dish, I would recommend 1 tablespoon per person. Plate and garnish with cilantro leaves. Serve with white rice and enjoy!

COCO-PASSION FRUIT CBD POPSICLES *with* PINEAPPLE *and* WILD RASPBERRY

During the peak of summer when you're craving something cold, surprise your friends with this tasty indulgence. This CBD popsicle recipe is almost as good as your next island getaway! Tropical fruits are the theme for this recipe, and I couldn't think of a more perfect addition than CBD coconut oil. The flavors blend perfectly to create this low-dose frosty treat.

SERVINGS: 6 popsicles	**TARGET DOSE:** 9 mg CBD | 0.67 mg THC per pop (using CBD Coconut Oil, page 63) or 11 mg CBD per pop (using commercially made CBD oil, see note below)

EQUIPMENT
Blender
Measuring cups
Measuring spoons
Standing popsicle mold kit
Popsicle sticks
4" x 6" (10 x 15 cm) cellophane bags

½ cup (65 g) fresh raspberries

1 tablespoon (15 ml) fresh lemon juice

½ cup (85 g) pineapple chunks

½ cup (120 ml) passion fruit juice (preferably not from concentrate)

2 tablespoons (30 ml) liquified CBD Coconut Oil (page 63)

¾ cup (175 ml) canned cream of coconut

¾ cup (175 ml) unsweetened coconut milk

Add the raspberries, lemon juice, pineapple, passion fruit juice, and CBD coconut oil to a blender. Blend, then empty the mixture into a clean container, and set aside.

Clean your blender, then blend the cream of coconut and coconut milk together. Set aside. Divide the CBD–fruit juice mixture evenly into 6 popsicle molds. Note: this is the infused portion, so spreading evenly is key! Layer the coconut cream milk on top. Insert 6 popsicle sticks and freeze overnight.

The next day, remove the pops from the molds. To do this, fill a mug with warm water and then dip each mold into the warmed water for a few seconds to help slide the popsicles out. Place them into cellophane bags and then store in a zip-top freezer bag. Immediately wash the molds and create another batch, if needed.

NOTE *If you don't have time to make your own CBD coconut oil, you can still incorporate CBD into this recipe by adding your favorite commercially made CBD oil. Simply mix 2 droppers full (66 mg CBD) of unflavored CBD oil of your choice (preferably made with coconut MCT oil) with 1 tablespoon plus 2½ teaspoons (26 ml) regular liquified coconut oil, then add to the recipe as directed.*

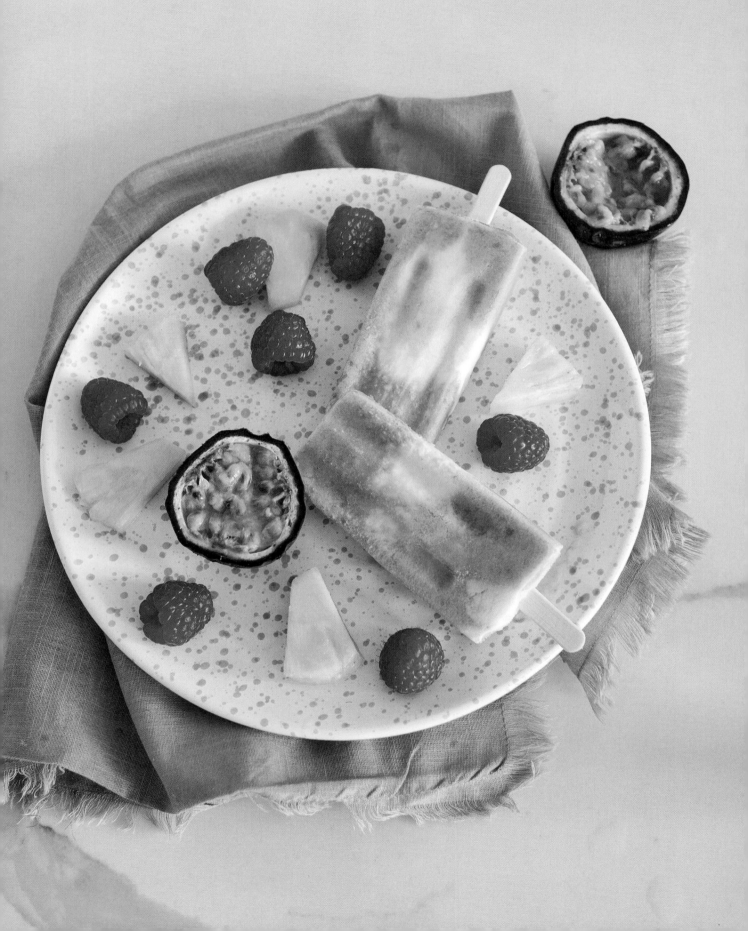

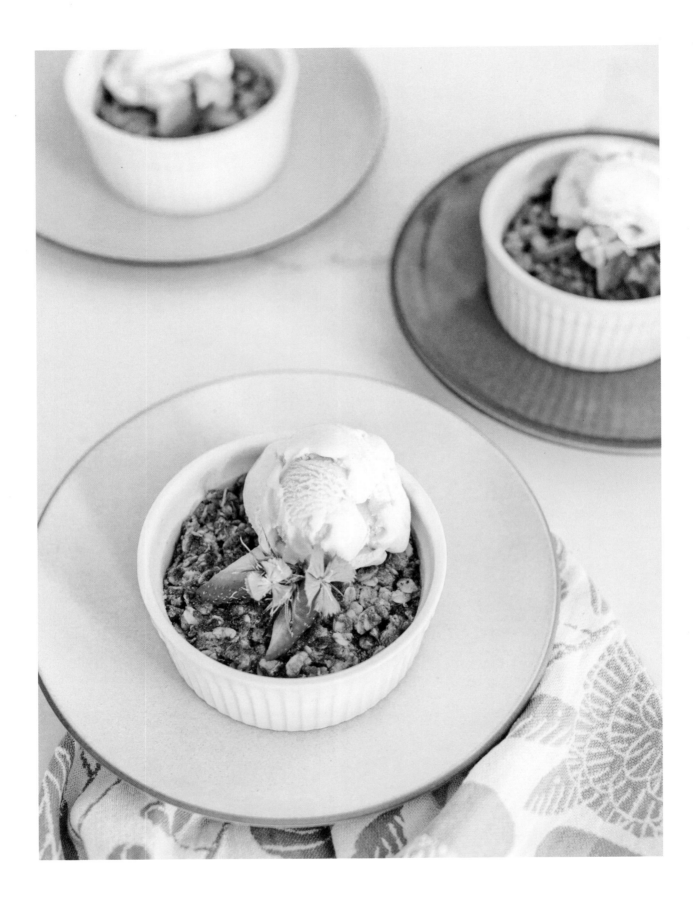

STRAWBERRY PEACH CBD CRISP

If you love dessert, this strawberry peach CBD crisp is the recipe you've been waiting for! If you're not the best at baking, don't worry. Crisps are incredibly easy to assemble, making this a perfect CBD baked dessert for you to experiment with. Top this recipe with a scoop of vanilla ice cream, and garnish with a slice of strawberry and peach. It's too delicious to pass up!

YIELD: **4** servings	**TARGET DOSE:** 13 mg CBD | 0.87 mg THC per crisp (using CBD-Rich Flower Butter, page 64) or 13 mg CBD per crisp (using CBD Isolate Butter, page 65) *includes estimated 13 percent loss of CBD and THC from baking in the oven

EQUIPMENT

Four 6-ounce (177 ml) porcelain ramekin baking dishes
Measuring cups
Measuring spoons
Mixing bowl
Small saucepan

STRAWBERRY PEACH FILLING

1½ cups (255 g) fresh strawberries, diced

1½ cups (255 g) fresh peaches, peeled and diced (can substitute for frozen if not in season)

½ cup (100 g) granulated sugar

2 tablespoons (30 ml) fresh lemon juice

GRANOLA CRISP TOPPING

4 tablespoons (55 g) salted butter

2 tablespoons (28 g) CBD butter of your choice (pages 64 and 65)

1 cup (96 g) oats

1 cup (120 g) whole-grain oat flour

½ cup (75 g) unpacked brown sugar

¾ teaspoon ground cinnamon

¾ teaspoon ground nutmeg

TOPPINGS (optional)

4 scoops vanilla ice cream

Strawberry and peach slices

Preheat the oven to 350°F (177°C). Spray the ramekins with cooking spray and set aside.

To make the filling: In a medium bowl, stir together the strawberries, peaches, granulated sugar, and lemon juice. Mix well and spoon into the ramekins. Set aside.

To make the topping: In a small saucepan, soften the salted butter and CBD butter together. Stir until blended well. Remove from the heat and add the oats, flour, brown sugar, cinnamon, nutmeg. Mix with a fork until crumbly.

Using your hands, pat the granola crisp mixture on top of the fruit mixture and spread evenly. Bake for 30 to 40 minutes, or until the crust is golden brown and crispy and the filling is bubbling. Top with a scoop of vanilla ice cream and a few sliced strawberries and peaches before serving, as desired.

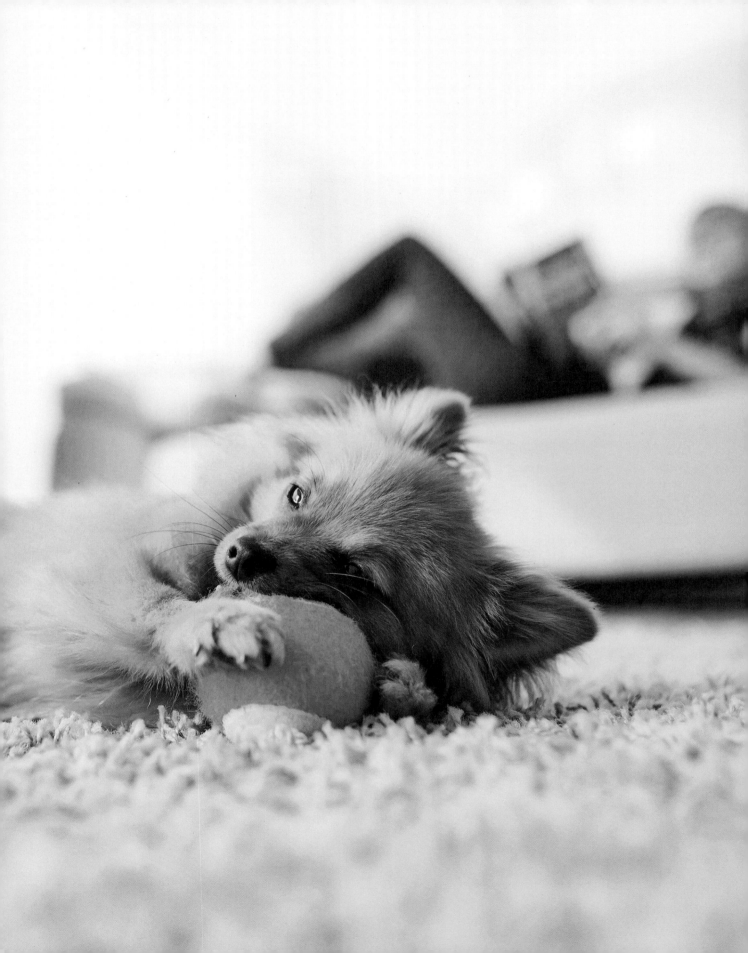

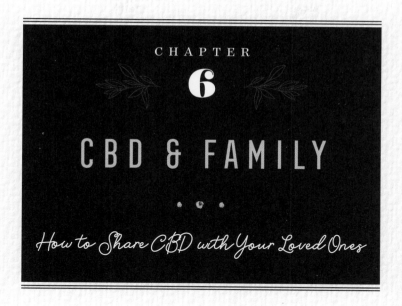

CHAPTER

6

CBD & FAMILY

• • •

How to Share CBD with Your Loved Ones

While learning how to integrate CBD into your daily routines and rit-uals, you might want to share the journey with the ones you love the most, family. Whether you are thinking about exploring CBD for your parents, your child, or for a pet, this chapter will help you determine if cannabidiol is a good fit for your loved ones.

As you've learned, CBD is derived from cannabis or hemp. While it might seem scary or intimidating when thinking about giving it to others, particularly children and pets, remember that responsibly sourced and produced CBD is a safe, nonintoxicating compound. When admin-istered correctly, it can potentially deliver therapeutic effects to help aid many health issues.

Before sharing CBD with your family, you might also encounter some family members that stigmatize anything having to do with cannabis, particularly parents or grandparents that lived through the "Reefer Madness" era. While cannabis and hemp products are becoming more mainstream these days, it can still be difficult to approach the subject if someone in your family has strong opposing feelings. The best way to end the stigma is by gently educating your loved ones. This chapter will provide you with talking points that can help you with these potentially challenging conversations.

Remember, cannabis is a natural botanical. It has been used for centuries to treat different ailments, so don't be afraid to share it with your family if you think it will benefit them.

6 THINGS YOUR FAMILY MEMBERS SHOULD KNOW ABOUT CBD

The first step to successfully introducing CBD to your family—even if it's just you that will be using CBD products—is to help those closest to you better understand how and why CBD can benefit the body and mind. Although every household is different, here are six things your family should know.

CBD Comes from a Plant

Okay, this might seem obvious, but, at the end of the day, it's good to remind your family members that CBD is an all-natural substance that comes from a plant, cannabis. Cannabis is a botanical that can heal us. It's not about getting stoned; it's about getting healthy.

CBD Isolates Won't Get You High, But Full-Spectrum Is the Best Medicine

CBD on its own will not get you or anyone in your family high or stoned. Whether you are giving cannabidiol to a child, pet, or parent, isolated cannabidiol does not produce any intoxicating effects; however, as you've learned, taking CBD on its own is not the optimal way to utilize it medicinally. Instead, it's best to educate your family on the benefits of using full-spectrum CBD containing varying levels of THC and other cannabinoids and terpenes, which enhance the efficacy of cannabidiol. Before administering to family members, be sure to know what ratios are in the product and stick to a 20:1 or 18:1 (CBD to THC) ratio, if you're looking to avoid THC's euphoria. To avoid THC altogether, which is best for pets and some family members, look for broad-spectrum hemp-derived CBD products.

CBD Can Help Parents Become More Patient and Present

Let's face it, being a parent is hard work. Whether you are experiencing a lack of sleep, stress, or irritability, CBD can help take the edge off and help you be more patient and present with your little ones. Some parents are even giving up their anti-anxiety medications as they are finding cannabidiol to be a more natural solution that doesn't impair the mind when taking care of the kids.

CBD is Safe for Children Who Need It

Adults aren't the only ones who can benefit from CBD's therapeutic effects. Children can benefit, too, particularly those who are living with epilepsy. Despite the lack of cannabis research, extensive studies have been done to examine cannabidiol as an effective treatment for reducing or stopping seizures in children with Dravet or Lennox-Gastaut syndrome. Because CBD is nonaddictive, nonintoxicating, and has a low risk of side effects, CBD is a hopeful solution that might also help children who suffer from autism and anxiety. If you're considering CBD for your child, be sure to consult with your pediatrician to figure out a plan that works best for their overall care, and keep them under close supervision during their treatments to watch for side effects. Turn to page 192 to learn more.

Hemp-Derived CBD Is Safe for Pets

Just like humans, animals have endocannabinoid systems that interact with phytocannabinoids to maintain homeostasis in the body. As a pet owner, you can safely integrate CBD into your dog or cat's health regimen to help with chronic pain, inflammation, autoimmune diseases, and more; however, animals metabolize CBD differently (i.e., dogs metabolize CBD differently than humans, and cats differently than dogs, etc.). *Be aware: THC can be toxic to pets.* It's best to stick with hemp-derived CBD products for your furry friends. See page 195 for more.

CBD Can Benefit Seniors

Due to CBD's soothing abilities and nonintoxicating side effects, cannabidiol is becoming a new tool that seniors are including in their health regimen, particularly those with arthritis, inflammation, sleep apnea, chronic pain, and anxiety. However, despite the many beneficial properties of CBD, it might not be a good fit for everyone due to the way it can interact with other medications. If you're thinking of using CBD for the first time, or you want to share CBD with someone in your household, be sure to consult with your doctor to ensure it's a safe choice. Flip to page 201 for a deeper look into CBD and senior care.

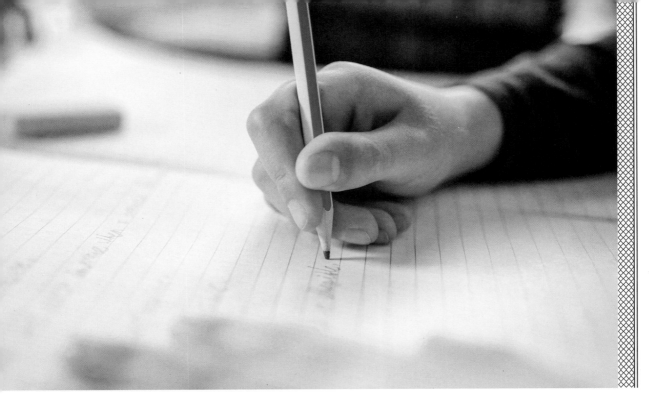

CBD could potentially be a solution for treating children with autism and anxiety, leading to a happier and healthier life.

CBD & CHILDREN

Treating your child with CBD is a choice that every parent should have the right to make. Traditional medicine and pharmaceutical drugs don't always work, especially for some of the most challenging conditions, making products made from cannabis and hemp a good alternative. If you believe that CBD might help your child, be sure to do your research, seek out a knowledgeable health care professional that specializes in cannabinoid medicine to ask questions, and find a reliable brand that produces clean products. Every child should have the chance to try various options for treatment, especially when facing a chronic disease or illness.

PRECAUTIONS & SIDE EFFECTS

After you've consulted with your pediatrician and feel good about your child's treatment plan, there are some precautions to take before giving CBD to kids. First of all, you'll want to source the best CBD possible. This can be a challenge as there are many, many brands that have jumped on the CBD bandwagon that have skipped getting their products tested for safety all together. While some of these less expensive options might seem enticing, by using untested products you could be exposing your child to pesticides or dangerous solvents, such as rubbing alcohol. Be sure to do your research.

If you're planning to explore THC as part of your child's medical care, seek the guidance of a trained health care professional. For children battling cancer or other serious health issues, THC is a viable option that many consider integrating into their existing health care plan. Due to the entourage effect, many of these patients are finding the best success using a balanced combination of CBD and THC as the two work synergistically for pain, inflammation, appetite, nausea, and more. However, be aware that THC has been known to negatively impact the developing adolescent brain. Only you can weigh the risks versus benefits and choose what's best for your young one.

When using plant medicine, the biggest challenge is finding the right dose, which might take some time as you experiment. Remember, everyone is different. Effects can vary drastically based on the child's age, weight and metabolism, the delivery method of CBD (or in some cases, THC), and the dosage the child is exposed to.

While CBD has few adverse side effects, the most commonly reported effects are tiredness, diarrhea, and changes in appetite and weight.

DELIVERY METHODS & PRODUCTS SUITABLE FOR CHILDREN

If you're considering CBD for your child, it is very important to do so under the close supervision of a pediatrician. For treatment, wellness physician and medical cannabis expert, Dr. Shivani Amin, recommends looking into oral delivery methods, such as tinctures, to deliver the medicine. Any child that she's treated with CBD or medical cannabis has always used tinctures as their primary product, where drops are taken underneath the tongue. Before administering, speak with a doctor and make sure that the CBD is not going to enhance or inhibit other medications that your child might be taking. Be smart, be proactive, and forget the stigma.

CBD: ALTERNATIVE MEDICINE FOR ADULTS & CHILDREN

featuring Dr. Shivani Amin, wellness physician & medical cannabis expert

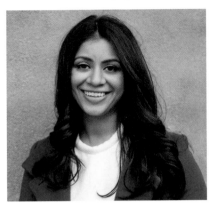

Dr. Shivani Amin specializes in functional medicine as a means to help her patients live more efficient lives without the debilitating side effects of pharmaceutical medications. She holds a strong passion for helping people live vibrantly through the practice of holistic and integrative medicine. Dr. Shivani is a leading authority on the responsible use of cannabis, CBD oil, and nutraceuticals. Focused on helping patients get to the root cause of their medical condition, Dr. Shivani strives to help patients achieve a unified mind-body-spirit connection as the pathway to optimal health and well-being. Follow Dr. Shivani Amin @drshivaniamin or visit www.drshivaniamin.com.

Dr. Shivani Amin: "Given my Indian ethnicity, I grew up surrounded by plants and herbs. As a child, my grandmother would always give me some form of herbal medicine when I was sick, and they always seemed to work! I, therefore, have always had it in my blood to embrace and practice more alternative medicine, which provoked me to start my cannabis clinics.

Throughout my practice, I have seen CBD benefit many people including adults and children. Some of the common conditions that I've treated are chronic pain, insomnia, seizures, and anxiety. Cannabidiol works well with our bodies because of our endocannabinoid systems (ECS). As a reminder, the ECS is a network of cell receptors, molecules, and enzymes found in the nervous system and brain. They work together to perform specific functions that include playing a role in pain sensation, mood, memory, and psychological processes.

CBD is a great solution for those looking for a natural path for healing. If you're thinking about using CBD for medical purposes, be aware that dosing is individually dependent and so is the delivery method—it really depends on what condition is being treated and the onset of medication. Whether you are looking to use CBD for yourself, or to treat a parent or child, remember that every patient is different. I cannot emphasize enough how important it is to speak with a knowledgeable health care provider about CBD and cannabis, especially if you're considering alternative medicine for serious health issues. Don't be afraid to ask questions. CBD and cannabis can heal countless chronic conditions, and with more research, education, and activism, I think we'll continue to see more and more health care professionals integrate alternative medicine into their practices."

CBD & PET CARE

If you've ever welcomed a pet into your life, you know how strong the emotional connection can be. Pets are considered part of the family, which means their health should be a priority. While many veterinarians are still in the early stages of using CBD for treatment, there's a growing number who are beginning to integrate cannabidiol into their practice now that there's research and reliable hemp-derived CBD products that have been developed specifically for dogs and cats. While CBD is picking up momentum, be aware that *THC is not safe for pets.* For this reason, pet owners are increasingly looking to hemp products as an option to help with pain management and much more.

The human and animal endocannabinoid system is very similar. Cannabinoid medicine researcher, Dr. Michele Ross, reports that our pets have the same major components of the endocannabinoid system, including CB1 and CB2 receptors, endocannabinoid anandamide (AEA) and 2-AG, and so on. Because CBD is an antioxidant that reduces pain, inflammation, and anxiety, it can be a great option for pet care. It's done wonders for older pets with arthritis and for pets recovering from surgery; however, it's not just for "sick" pets. Even the healthiest pets can benefit from CBD, which can help prevent endocannabinoid deficiencies that cause disease, Dr. Ross explains. Most of our pets are eating food that is lacking complete nutrition for physical and mental health. A daily CBD regimen can help restore balance to their endocannabinoid system and may reduce the need for prescription medications now or in the future as the pet ages.

Gillian Levy, master herbalist and co-founder of Humboldt Apothecary, produces a line of pet care products that are especially helpful for animals that experience anxiety. CBD oils can be used while traveling with your animal, during holidays like the Fourth of July (where there are frequent loud and frightening noises), or for everyday use to reduce general anxiety. Additionally, CBD can be useful for chronic inflammatory conditions, such as arthritis. Many people have reported that using CBD for arthritis can greatly increase the mobility of the animal, and can significantly improve the quality of their life.

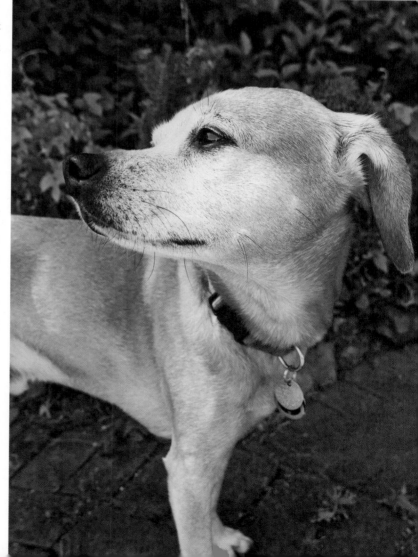

When administering CBD to your pet, like my dog Jameson here, remember the golden rule: "Start low, go slow." Titrate the dose up or down until the desired effect is achieved.

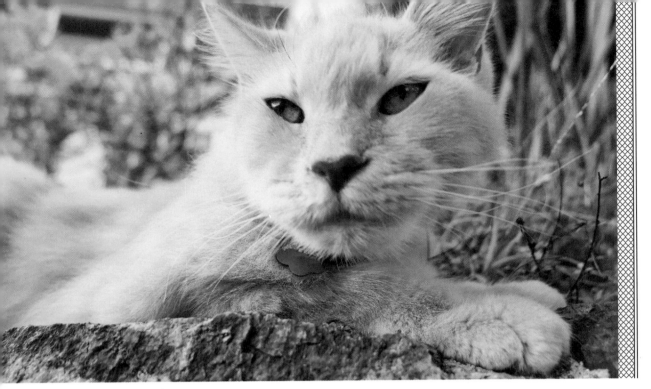

Remember, cats like Ollie here and dogs metabolize CBD differently. Speak with your veterinarian to figure out a dosing plan that works best for your animal companion.

CBD FOR DOGS VERSUS CATS

Whether you have a dog or cat, the process of treating your animal with CBD varies greatly from species to species. While all mammals contain endocannabinoid systems, they are not exactly the same. For instance, dogs have a higher concentration of endocannabinoid receptors in their cerebellum and brainstem (compared to humans and cats), which affects their coordination and heart rate. Due to these heightened levels of receptors, if a dog ingests a product that contains THC, the results can be toxic.

When it comes to cats, Amanda Howland, the co-founder of ElleVet Sciences, explains that your feline friends are not similar to small dogs. The half-life of medication in cats is very short, much shorter than that of dogs, so dosing CBD is quite different. Partnering with Cornell University's Veterinary School, ElleVet Sciences conducted the pharmacokinetic studies and research needed to understand how CBD is metabolized by dogs and cats. Through these studies, which were focused on pets with chronic pain, they were able to identify the accuracy and frequency of dosing. Ideally, when treating cats for chronic pain, they should be dosed multiple times per day. This might not be realistic for some cat owners, so a higher dose of 2 mg/kg twice a day is what is recommended, depending on the cat's needs. Dogs, on the other hand, typically need CBD supplements twice daily at 1 mg/kg to help with pain.

DELIVERY METHODS & PET CARE PRODUCTS

The delivery methods for administering CBD to pets is more simplified than it is for humans. The two most common and safe methods include oral delivery and topical use. While I shouldn't have to say it, pets should never be exposed to smoke or second-hand smoke as a way to administer CBD!

Oral Delivery

The most common method for administering CBD orally for pets is via hemp-derived CBD oils/tinctures and CBD pet treats. CBD oils can be taken directly through the mouth or they can be mixed into pet food, depending on what your pet prefers. Gillian Levy prefers tinctures because they are ideal for customizing a dose for a pet. Most pets seem to find the flavor palatable and by putting the drops directly into their food, you can streamline the precision of dosing based on the individual needs of the animal. CBD oils are best for pets that have food allergies or skin sensitivities, but because they do contain olive oil or coconut oil, your pet could experience diarrhea from extra oil being added into their diet. That said, CBD pet treats are a popular option, particularly for dogs. Turn to page 199 for a Gluten-Free CBD Peanut Butter Dog Treat recipe.

Topicals

Topicals are an excellent solution for pets to help manage joint inflammation, arthritis, scratches, and other minor skin irritations. It's often difficult to administer oral medications to felines, and studies are also suggesting that topicals might be the best application option for cats if applied inside the ear. For optimal results, look for broad-spectrum hemp CBD topicals that contain a range of cannabinoids (everything but THC) plus beneficial terpenes. See Resources on page 206 for a recommended product.

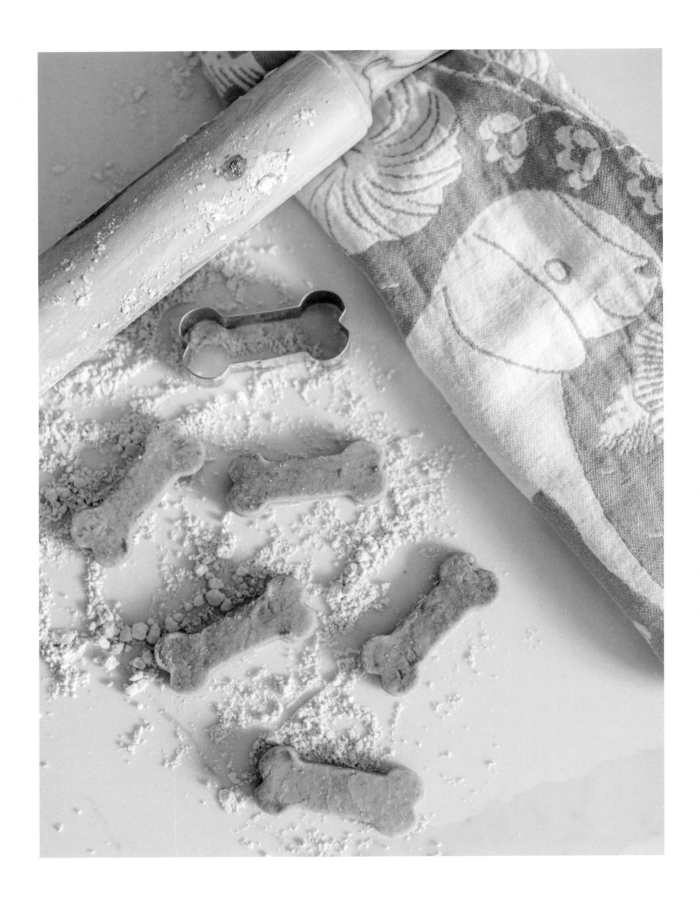

GLUTEN-FREE CBD PEANUT BUTTER DOG TREATS

If you enjoy creating treats for your furry friends at home, this gluten-free recipe will keep your pet smiling. This recipe is meant to contain 2 milligrams of CBD per biscuit. Depending on your dog's needs, you can either split this treat in half for a lower dose or give your dog a couple of treats if they require more. Also, be aware that your dog could have allergies to some of the ingredients listed. If this is a worry, check in with your veterinarian before serving.

YIELD: 37 to 38 treats	**TARGET DOSE:** 2 mg CBD per treat

EQUIPMENT
Baking sheet
Parchment paper
Electric hand mixer
2½-inch (6-cm) doggie bone cookie cutters
Measuring cups
Mixing bowls
Mixing spoon
Rolling pin

½ cup (125 g) unsweetened applesauce

3 droppers full hemp CBD pet oil (75 mg CBD)

½ cup (130 g) creamy, unsalted peanut butter

1 egg

6 tablespoons (90 ml) chicken stock

3 cups (360 g) oat flour

Preheat the oven to 350°F (177°C). Line a baking sheet with parchment paper.

Combine the applesauce and hemp CBD oil in a small bowl. Mix well with a spoon.

In a large mixing bowl, combine the CBD applesauce, peanut butter, egg, and chicken stock. Mix all ingredients using an electric hand mixer. Make sure to blend well so that the CBD distributes evenly. Once mixed well, slowly add the flour. Add 1 cup (120 g) at a time, mix, and then add the next. The dough will become thick and sticky. Use your hands to roll the dough into a ball.

Put the dough between two sheets of parchment paper and begin to roll it out using a rolling pin until the dough is flat, but still thick. Use your 2½-inch (6-cm) doggie bone cookie cutter to cut the treats, and place them onto a lined baking sheet. Continue to roll out the dough and cut treats until the dough is gone.

Bake for about 12 to 15 minutes and let cool before serving.

FINDING SAFE & RELIABLE CBD PRODUCTS FOR PETS

featuring Amanda Howland, Co-Founder & CBO, ElleVet Sciences

Amanda Howland is the co-founder and CBO of ElleVet Sciences, a leading maker of cannabinoid-based soft chews and CBD oil for pets. Amanda and her team develop hemp CBD pet products that are based on the science and data of research that they've conducted with Cornell University. Before co-founding ElleVet with her partner Christian Kjaer, Amanda worked in public health research. She has a BA from Colby College and a Masters in Public Health from the University of New England. She lives in Portland with her partner, three children, and two dogs. Follow Amanda and ElleVet Sciences @ellevetsciences.

Amanda Howland: "All mammals have endocannabinoid systems which are responsible for maintaining homeostasis within the body. There are receptors located throughout our central nervous system, peripheral nervous system, and the brain that interact with endocannabinoids and phytocannabinoids, which helps explain why CBD can aid many different diseases.

In the pharmacokinetic research that we've done at ElleVet, we've determined how CBD is metabolized by dogs and cats, which allows us to determine accurate dosing for different species. For example, based on our research and pharmacokinetic studies, a 1 mg/kg twice daily dose is the baseline to provide relief for dogs with chronic pain. Higher doses are appropriate for some disease areas.

As you've learned throughout this book, all CBD is not created equal. The same goes for pet CBD products. There are many poor-quality products out there, which means pet owners need to do their due diligence and dosing needs to be accurate. Most products we've seen are greatly underdosing and are made from inferior resources, which isn't going to give your pet the help it needs. As a general rule, look for full-spectrum or broad-spectrum (i.e., CBD products that contain a wide range of cannabinoids and a robust terpene profile), a high mg/ml potency, a Certificate of Analysis (COA) for every batch, or a product that has been tested in a clinical trial by a university or accredited institution. These are all basic criteria that should be met by any reputable company.

When administering CBD to a pet, it is extremely safe, but be sure the product *does not* contain THC in amounts higher than 0.3% by weight as THC can be toxic, particularly to dogs. That said, if you're considering giving CBD to your pet, be open to speaking with your veterinarian about CBD treatment. We work with vets from all over the country and have found that they are extremely accepting and supportive of using high-quality and well-tested CBD products. Veterinarians like ElleVet because of our research as well as ongoing clinical trials that are science and data focused.

Overall, CBD is a wonderful treatment method for pets and can change the face of pain management in veterinary medicine when used properly. Ask us or ask your vet—don't be afraid to ask questions. Be an advocate for your animal!"

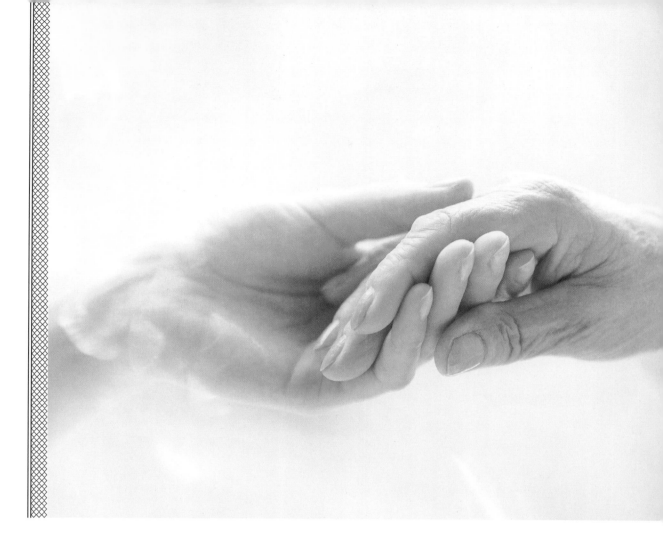

CBD & SENIORS

Seniors are increasingly turning to CBD as a wellness tool, as it can provide relief for anxiety, arthritis, pain relief, and more without compromising mental clarity. Seniors are loving CBD so much, that they are quickly becoming one of the fastest growing demographics of people who are using cannabis and hemp-derived CBD products.

Okay, you may be thinking, "Really? My grandma would never use cannabis products." That is a common reaction due to the era many senior patients grew up in (i.e., the early days of prohibition and the War on Drugs, where cannabis was demonized). Now that there is more and more research and science-backed studies coming out, I think you'd be surprised about how curious your grandma might be about trying CBD. Also, guess what? Many seniors are letting go of those old stigmas because they are finding personal success using cannabidiol.

It all comes down to education. If you're thinking about giving CBD to a parent or grandparent, be sure to sit down with them and spend some time explaining how cannabidiol works with the endocannabinoid system and the ways in which CBD can benefit them.

PRECAUTIONS

If you're a senior reading this book, or otherwise considering giving CBD to a parent, be sure to check in with a health care professional and let them know that you're considering using CBD. This is especially important if other medications are involved. As you learned from Dr. Michele Ross on page 30, CBD is a potent inhibitor of two types of p450 liver and gut enzymes that break down over a third of prescription drugs. If you're using CBD with a drug that is metabolized by enzymes such as CYP3A4, CBD can affect how long the drug will stay in your system, which can cause amplified side effects. Pay close attention to warning labels on medication bottles. As a rule of thumb, if a medication says, "Do Not Consume with Grapefruit," you should probably not be taking CBD with that medication either (CBD and grapefruit are known to interact with similar drugs based on those enzymes).

DELIVERY METHODS & BEST PRODUCTS FOR SENIORS

For the most part, CBD is very safe for senior patients and can be tolerated in higher doses if approved by a health care professional. Here is a brief overview of the most common delivery methods and products for senior care.

Oral Delivery

Oral consumption delivery methods, such as tinctures, are a great option for senior care as they deliver precise dosing as well as allow you to titrate doses either up or down depending on the individual's needs. In Dr. Shivani Amin's practice, senior patients mostly work with tinctures for this reason. CBD sublingual strips are also a fast and efficient option for relief. Simply put a strip under the tongue, let it dissolve, and effects should kick in within 15 to 45 minutes. Low-dose THC edibles are another option for senior care; however, depending on the person and their medical condition, a higher dose of THC might be required to best deal with pain or other intended benefits.

Topicals

Topicals are extremely approachable for seniors who are brand new to cannabis or hemp-based products. They provide a first step toward discovering the many ways that CBD and cannabinoid-based medicine can work with the body. Lotions, balms, and salves are all great options for care as the CBD is absorbed through the skin to target areas such as sore hands due to arthritis. Topicals containing THC are especially effective for those looking for pain relief and will not deliver any intoxicating side effects, no matter how much is applied to the skin. Turn to page 74 for a deeper look into topicals, other self-care products, and how to use them.

Transdermal Patches

CBD transdermal patches are a great solution for seniors who are looking for whole-body, long-lasting relief. Unlike CBD creams, balms, and salves, the heat activated transdermal patch will release small amounts of CBD through the skin and into your bloodstream, circulating throughout your entire body. Transdermal delivery releases CBD slowly over a number of hours with effects lasting up to 12 hours depending on the potency of the patch. If you're using a patch that contains both CBD and THC, you'll most likely not feel enhanced psycho-active effects, but know that THC will be going into your bloodstream.

To use, choose a place on your body that is free of hair and not oily such as the inside of your wrist, inside or outside of your bicep, under your armpit or on top of your foot. Clean the area with an alcohol swab and dry thoroughly before applying the patch. Onset times can vary, but expect to feel some relief within 1 hour to 1½ hours. You can also use in conjunction with other CBD topicals if you'd like to.

HEALING CBD HAND SALVE

If you or a loved one struggles with arthritis, this CBD-rich healing hand salve is a great recipe to make at home. Combining the soothing powers of CBD coconut oil, arnica, and frankincense, this therapeutic combination can help relieve sore joints, pain, and swelling in the hands, plus heal dry cuticles. Arnica is also a powerful remedy that can help heal bruises and frankincense helps reduce inflammation. Use this hand salve daily for best results.

YIELD: 4½ to 5 ounces (130 to 140 g)	**TARGET DOSE:** 224 mg CBD | 16 mg THC per batch (using CBD Coconut Oil [page 63]) or 333 mg CBD per batch (using commercially made CBD oil, see note below)

EQUIPMENT

One 8-ounce (240-ml) sterilized
   Mason jar
Measuring cup
Measuring spoons
Small saucepan
Spoon
Oven mitt

½ cup (120 ml) CBD Coconut Oil
   (page 63; see note)

2 heaping tablespoons (20 g) beeswax
   pellets

2 teaspoons (10 ml) argan oil

10 drops arnica oil

10 drops frankincense essential oil

In the Mason jar, combine the CBD coconut oil and beeswax.

Fill up a small saucepan about halfway with water. Place the *unsealed* Mason jar inside and begin to heat on low. Gently stir the mixture until both the beeswax and CBD coconut oil have fully melted.

Remove from the heat. Quickly combine with the argan, arnica, and frankincense oils, and then stir the CBD mixture. At this point, you can transfer the salve to a different storage container or keep it in your Mason jar.

Seal with an airtight lid and let cool. For storage, keep your CBD hand salve in a cool location where it will remain semi-solid. To use, simply use your fingernail to remove the salve from the jar, and massage into the hands for relief.

NOTE | *To substitute professionally made CBD oil into this recipe, simply use regular coconut oil when heating. Skip the argan oil and replace with 2 teaspoons (10 ml) of unflavored CBD oil of your choice (preferably made with fractionated coconut or MCT oil), then follow the directions as written.*

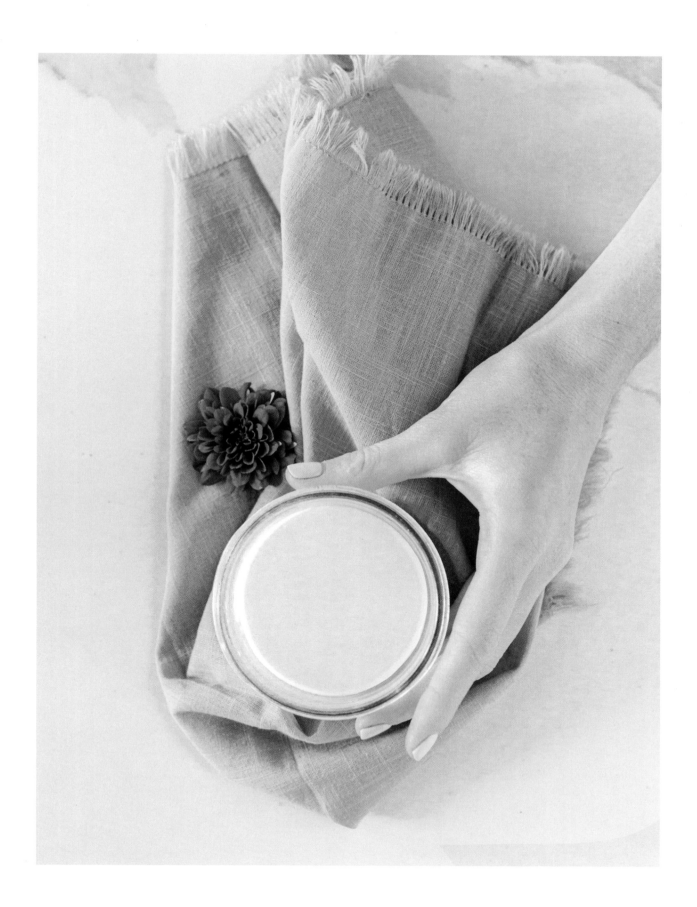

RESOURCES

CBD ISOLATES

CBD Distillery 99%+ Pure CBDelicious
Formulation Powder

CBD Distillery 99+% Pure CBD Isolate Powder
(Crystalline)

DRY FLOWER VAPORIZER

Firefly 2 Vaporizer from Firefly

CBD TINCTURES

Humboldt Apothecary CBD Tinctures

Juna

ONDA Wellness

Papa & Barkley Essentials Hemp Drops and Product Line

CBD BEAUTY PRODUCTS

Kiskanu Beauty Products

Saint Jane

Vertly Lip Balm

Vertly Bath Salts

Vertly Workout Recovery Body Spray

CBD INTIMATE PRODUCTS

Quim Happy Clam Everyday Oil

Quim Night Moves Intimate Oil

Quim OH Yes! Latex-Safe Serum

EDIBLE PRODUCTS

Garden Society

Kiva Confections

INFUSION DEVICES

Nova by Ardent

LEVO II Oil Infusion Device

The MagicalButter Machine

PET CARE

ElleVet Sciences Hemp CBD Chews & Hemp CBD Oil—
Feline and Canine

Treatibles Broad-Spectrum Hemp Oil Topical
Cream 240 mg—Feline and Canine

READY-TO-USE GOURMET CBD PRODUCTS

Pot d'Huile Olive Oil

Potli Honey and Infused Panty Items

Mondo THC and CBD Powder

TRUSTED VAPORIZERS

Bloom Farms

Chemistry

Care by Design

TSO Sonoma

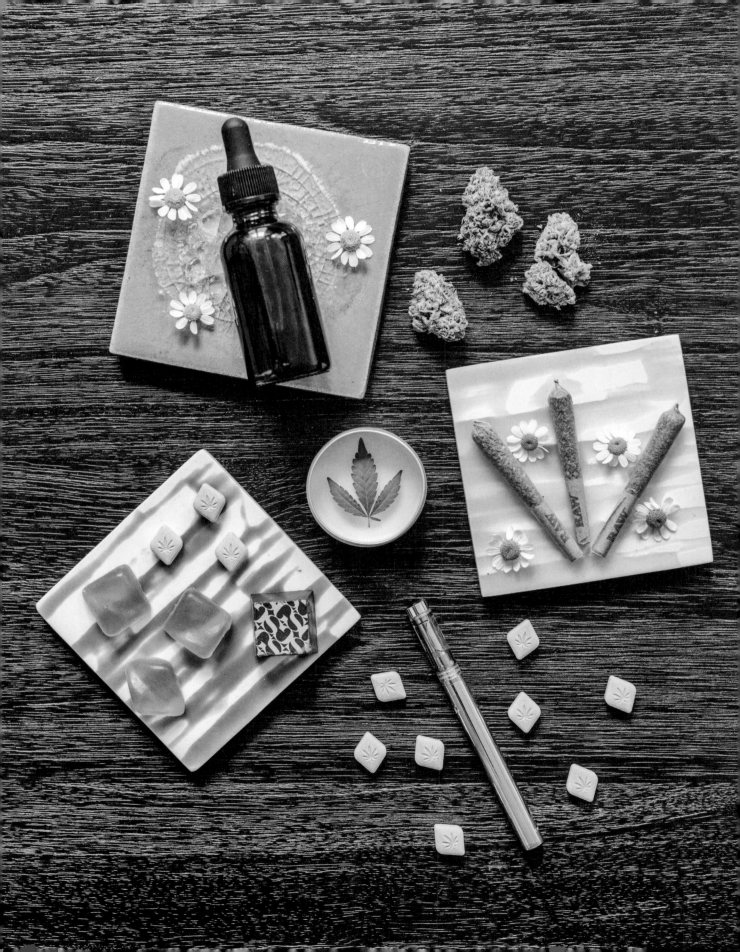

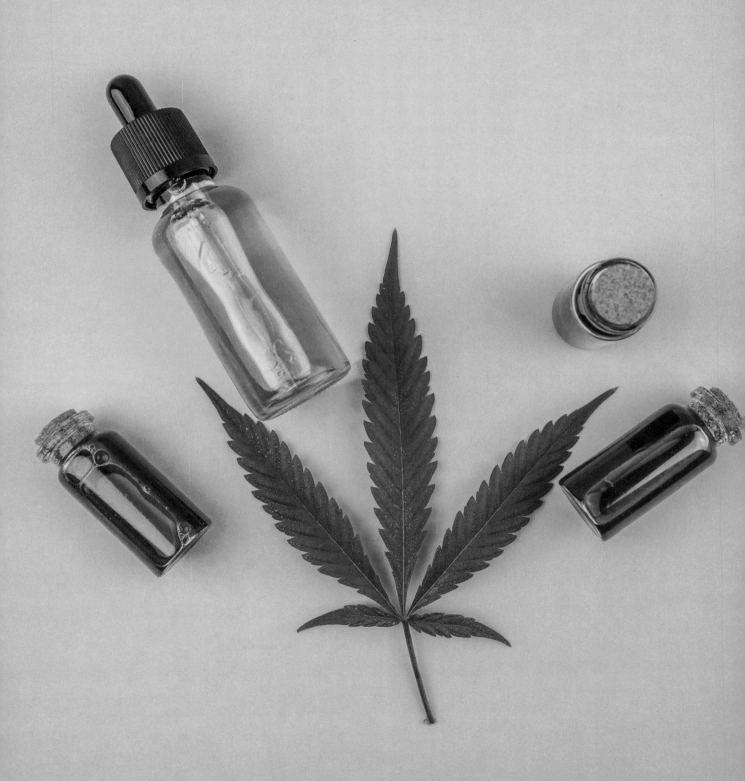

WORKS CITED

CHAPTER 1: GETTING STARTED WITH CBD

Abazia, D. et al. "Reefer Madness or Real Medicine? A Plea for Incorporating Medicinal Cannabis in Pharmacy Curricula." *Currents in Pharmacy Teaching and Learning.* September 2018.

Apostu, D. et al. "Cannabinoids and Bone Regeneration." *Drug Metabolism Review.* February 2019.

Barrus, D. et al. "Tasty THC: Promises and Challenges of Cannabis Edibles." *Methods Report RTI Press.* November 2016.

Boggs, D. et al. "Clinical and Preclinical Evidence for Functional Interactions of Cannabidiol and 9-Tetrahydrocannabinol." *Neuropyschopharmacology.* January 2018.

Bolognini, D. et al. "Cannabidiolic Acid Prevents Vomiting in Suncus Murinus and Nausea-Induced Behaviour in Rats by Enhancing 5-HT1A Receptor Activation." *British Journal of Pharmacology.* March 2013.

Chye, Y. et al. "The Endocannabinoid System and Cannabidiol's Promise for the Treatment of Substance Use Disorder." *Front Psychiatry.* February 2019.

Corroon, J. et al. "The Endocannabinoid System and Its Modulation by Cannabidiol (CBD)." *Alternative Therapies in Health and Medicine.* June 2019.

Di Marzo, V. "Inhibitory Effect of Cannabichromene, a Major Non-Psychotropic Cannabinoid Extracted from Cannabis Sativa, On Inflammation-Induced Hypermotility in Mice." *British Journal of Pharmacology.* February 2012.

Hindocha, C. et al. "Acute Effects of Cannabinoids on Addiction Endophenotypes Are Moderated by Genes Encoding the CB1 Receptor and FAAH Enzyme." *Addiction Biology.* April 2019.

Huestis, M. et al. "Cannabidiol Adverse Effects and Toxicity." *Current Neuropharmacology.* June 2019.

Huestis, M. "Human Cannabinoid Pharmacokinetics." *Chemistry & Biodiversity.* August 2007.

Huizenga, M. et al. "Preclinical Safety and Efficacy of Cannabidivarin for Early Life Seizures." *Neuropharmocology.* April 2019.

Hurd, Y. et al. "Early Phase in the Development of Cannabidiol As a Treatment for Addiction: Opioid Relapse Takes Initial Center Stage." *Neurotherapeutics.* October 2015.

Iffland, K. et al. "An Update on Safety and Side Effects of Cannabidiol: A Review of Clinical Data and Relevant Animal Studies." *Cannabis and Cannabinoid Research*. June 2017.

Izzo, C. et al. "What Is the Endocannabinoid System and What Is Its Role?" *Leafly*. December 2016.

Kathmann, F. et al. "Cannabidiol Is an Allosteric Modulator at Mu- and Delta-Opioid Receptors." *Naunyn Schmiedebergs Archives of Pharmacology*. February 2006.

Kerr, S. "Managing Nausea with Cannabis." *Project CBD*. February 2018.

Lee, M. "The Endocannabinoid System" *Project CBD*.

Lee, M. "What Is CBD?" *Project CBD*.

Leinow, L. et al. *CBD: A Patient's Guide to Medicinal Cannabis*. North Atlantic Books, 2017.

Martin, R. et al. "Cognitive Functioning Following Long-Term Cannabidiol Use in Adults with Treatment-Resistant Epilepsy." *Epilepsy & Behavior*. June 2019.

Millar, S. et al. "A Systematic Review of Cannabidiol Dosing in Clinical Populations." *British Journal of Clinical Pharmacology*. June 2019.

Millar, S. et al. "A Systematic Review on the Pharmacokinetics of Cannabidiol in Humans." *Frontiers in Pharmacology*. November 2018.

Miziak, B. et al. "Drug-Drug Interactions Between Antiepileptics and Cannabinoids." *Expert Opinion on Drug Metabolism & Toxicology*. May 2019.

Modesto, N. et al. "Cannabis and Cannabinoids on Treatment of Inflammation: A Patent Review." *Recent Patents on Biotechnology*. June 2019.

Oláh, A. et al. "Differential Effectiveness of Selected Non-Psychotropic Phytocannabinoids on Human Sebocyte Functions Implicates Their Introduction in Dry/Seborrhoeic Skin and Acne Treatment." *Experimental Dermatology*. June 2016.

Osborne, A. et al. "Effect of Cannabidiol on Endocannabinoid, Glutamatergic, and Gabaergic Signaling Markers in Male Offspring of a Maternal Immune Activation (Poly I:C) Model Relevant to Schizophrenia." *Progress in Neuropsychopharmacology & Biological Psychiatry*. June 2019.

Palermino, C. "This Is How You Actually Dose CBD." *Nice Paper*. February 2019.

Ross, M. *Vitamin Weed: A 4-Step Plan to Prevent and Reverse Endocannabinoid Deficiency*. Green Stone Books, 2018.

Russo, E. "CBD, the Entourage Effect and the Microbiome" *Project CBD*. January 2019.

Russo, E. "Taming THC: Potential Cannabis Synergy and Phytocannabinoid-Terpenoid Entourage Effects." *British Journal of Pharmacology*. August 2011.

Shannon, S. "Effectiveness of Cannabidiol Oil for Pediatric Anxiety and Insomnia as Part of Posttraumatic Stress Disorder: A Case Report." *The Permanente Journal.* Fall 2016.

Shinjyo, N. et al. "The Effect of Cannabichromene on Adult Neural Stem/Progenitor Cells." *Neurochemistry International.* November 2013.

Welty, T. et al. "Cannabidiol: Promise and Pitfalls." *American Epilepsy Society.* September 2014.

White, C. "A Review of Human Studies Assessing Cannabidiol's (CBD) Therapeutic Actions and Potential." *Journal of Clinical Pharmacology.* July 2019.

Whyte, L. et al. "The Putative Cannabinoid Receptor GPR55 Affects Osteoclast Function in Vitro and Bone Mass In Vivo." *Proceedings of the National Academy of Sciences of the U S A.* September 2009.

Xu, C. et al. "Pharmacokinetics of Oral and Intravenous Cannabidiol and Its Antidepressant-Like Effects in Chronic Mild Stress Mouse Model." *Environmental Toxicology & Pharmacology.* May 2019.

CHAPTER 2: DIY WITH CBD

Booth, J. et al. "Terpene Synthases from Cannabis Sativa" *PLOS One.* March 2017.

Cervantes, J. *The Cannabis Encyclopedia.* Van Patten Publishing, 2015.

Editorial Staff. "17 Truly High CBD Strains and Their Effects (the Complete List)." *Green Camp.* December 2017.

Gallily, R. et al. "The Anti-Inflammatory Properties of Terpenoids from *Cannabis.*" *Cannabis and Cannabinoid Research.* December 2018.

Goldleaf Ltd. *The Cooking Journal: A Cannabis Culinary Companion.* Fairfield, OH: Goldleaf Ltd, 2018.

Kuhathasan, N. et al. "The Use of Cannabinoids for Sleep: A Critical Review on Clinical Trials." *Experimental and Clinical Psychopharmacology.* May 2019.

Lee, M. "Terpenes and the Entourage Effect." *Project CBD.*

Leinow, L. et al. *CBD: A Patient's Guide to Medicinal Cannabis.* Berkeley, CA: North Atlantic Books, 2018.

Mudge, E. et al. "The Terroir of Cannabis: Terpene Metabolomics as a Tool to Understand Cannabis Sativa Selections." *Planta Medica.* July 2019.

Nuutinen, T. et al. "Medicinal Properties of Terpenes Found in Cannabis Sativa and Humulus Lupulus." *European Journal of Medicinal Chemistry.* September 2018.

Ross, M. *Vitamin Weed: A 4-Step Plan to Prevent and Reverse Endocannabinoid Deficiency.* Green Stone Books, 2018.

Russo, E. "The Case for the Entourage Effect and Conventional Breeding of Clinical Cannabis: No 'Strain,' No Gain." *Frontiers in Plant Science*. January 2019.

Shannon, S. et al. "Cannabidiol in Anxiety and Sleep: A Large Case Series." *The Permanente Journal*. January 2019.

Solymosi, K. et al. "Cannabis: A Treasure Trove or Pandora's Box?" *Mini Reviews in Medicinal Chemistry*. 2017.

CHAPTER 3: CBD & SELF-CARE

Babson, K. et al. "Cannabis, Cannabinoids, and Sleep: A Review of the Literature." March 2017.

Douglas, S. "A Runner's Guide to CBD." *Runner's World*. September 2019.

Fetters, K. "Can CBD Products Improve Your Fitness Results?" *US News & World Report*. May 2018.

Hendricks, O. et al. "Efficacy and Safety of Cannabidiol Followed by an Open Label Add-On of Tetrahydrocannabinol for the Treatment of Chronic Pain in Patients with Rheumatoid Arthritis or Ankylosing Spondylitis: Protocol for a Multicentre, Randomized, Placebo-Controlled Study." *BMJ Open*. June 2019.

Jhawar, N. et al. "The Growing Trend of Cannabidiol in Skincare Products." *Clinics in Dermatology*. May–June 2019.

Kelly, E. "A Fit Person's Guide to CBD Products and Supplements." *GQ*. August 2018.

Kennedy, M. "Cannabis: Exercise Performance and Sport. A Systematic Review." *Journal of Science and Medicine in Sport*. March 2017.

Kubala, J. "7 Benefits and Uses of CBD Oil (Plus Side Effects)." *Healthline*. February 2018.

Lapidos, R. "Why Cannabis Is the Buzziest Ingredient in Skin Care." *Well and Good*. April 2018.

Oláh, A. et al. "Cannabidiol Exerts Sebostatic and Anti-Inflammatory Effects on Human Sebocytes." *The Journal of Clinical Investigation*. September 2014.

Palmieri, B. et al. "A Therapeutic Effect of CBD-Enriched Ointment in Inflammatory Skin Diseases and Cutaneous Scars." *La Clinica Terapeutica*. March–April 2017.

Ries, J. "Can CBD Improve Your Sex Life?" *Huffington Post*. September 2018.

Sangiovanni, E. et al. "Cannabis Sativa L. Extract and Cannabidiol Inhibit In Vitro Mediators of Skin Inflammation and Wound Injury." *Phytotherapy Research* June 2019.

Staff Writer. "How CBD Works" *Project CBD*. 2018.

CHAPTER 4: CBD & BEVERAGES

Bobrow, W. *Cannabis Cocktails, Mocktails & Tonics.* Beverly, MA: Quarto Publishing Group USA Inc., 2016.

Boudinot, J. "Cocktails with Chronic: How to Infuse Liquor with Weed." *Paste Magazine.* February 2017.

Chung, T. et al. "Cannabis and Alcohol: From Basic Science to Public Policy." *Alcohol Clinical and Experimental Research.* July 2019.

Dao, D. "CBD Cocktails: What They Are and Why They're Taking Over Bar Menus Everywhere." *Food & Wine Magazine.* October 2018.

De Ternay, J. et al. "Therapeutic Prospects of Cannabidiol for Alcohol Use Disorder and Alcohol-Related Damages on the Liver and the Brain." *Frontiers in Pharmacology.* May 2019.

Fernández-Ruiz, J. et al. "Cannabidiol for Neurodegenerative Disorders: Important New Clinical Applications for This Phytocannabinoid?" *British Journal of Clinical Pharmacology.* May 2012.

June-Wells, M. "Your Guide to Ethanol Extraction." *Cannabis Business Times.* July 2018.

Konen, B. "Part 4, How to Dose Homemade Cannabis Edibles." *Leafly.* April 2016.

Korkidis, J. "Fat-Washed Cannabis-Infused Alcohol." *Chron Vivant.* December 2017.

Lee, M. "Cannabis Dosing 101." *Project CBD.* May 2018.

Leinow, L. et al. *CBD: A Patient's Guide to Medical Cannabis.* Berkeley, CA: North Atlantic Books, 2017.

Magner, E. "What Really Happens When You Mix CBD and Alcohol." *Well Good.* September 2019.

Mark, K. "How Sunflower Lecithin May Help CBD Work Better and Faster." *2RiseNatural.* June 2017.

Nona, C. et al. "Effects of Cannabidiol on Alcohol-Related Outcomes: A Review of Preclinical and Human Research." *Experiments in Clinical Psychopharmacology.* May 2019.

Owram, K. "Scientists Are Racing to Make Weed as Easy to Drink as Beer." *Bloomberg.* February 2019.

Powers, D. "How to Make CBD Cocktails at Home." *Civilized.* September 2018.

Staff Writer. "11-Hydroxy-THC—Increased Potency That Explains the Effect of Edibles?" *Prof of Pot.* July 2019.

CHAPTER 5: CBD & COOKING

Editorial Staff. "17 Truly High CBD Strains and Their Effects (the Complete List)." *Green Camp.* December 2017.

Editorial Staff. "Top 10 Evidence-Based Health Benefits of Coconut Oil." *HealthLine.*

Goldleaf Ltd. *The Cooking Journal: A Cannabis Culinary Companion.* Fairfield, OH: Goldleaf Ltd, 2018.

Greenspan, D. *Butter.* Virginia, USA: Short Stack Editions, 2017.

Hua, S. et al. *Edibles: Small Bites for the Modern Cannabis Kitchen.* San Francisco, CA: Chronicle Books, 2018.

Jeff the 420 Chef. *The 420 Gourmet: The Elevated Art of Cannabis Cuisine.* New York, New York: Harper Collins Publishers, 2016.

Konen, B. "Part 4, How to Dose Homemade Cannabis Edibles." *Leafly.* April 2016.

McDonough, E. *Bong Appetit: Mastering the Art of Cooking with Weed.* Berkeley, CA: Ten Speed Press, 2018.

Sicard, C. "10 Common Marijuana Cooking Mistakes and How to Avoid Them." *Cannabis Cheri.* April 2018.

CHAPTER 6: CBD & FAMILY

Barchel, D. et al. "Oral Cannabidiol Use in Children with Autism Spectrum Disorder to Treat Related Symptoms and Co-Morbidities." *Frontiers in Pharmacololgy.* January 2019.

Chen, J. et al. "Cannabidiol: A New Hope for Patients with Dravet or Lennox-Gastaut Syndromes." *Annals of Pharmacotherapy.* June 2019.

Crippa, J. et al. "Translational Investigation of the Therapeutic Potential of Cannabidiol (CBD): Toward a New Age." *Frontiers in Immunology.* September 2018.

Gamble, L. et al. "Pharmacokinetics, Safety, and Clinical Efficacy of Cannabidiol Treatment in Osteoarthritic Dogs." *Frontiers.* July 2018.

Granta, I. et al. "Cannabis and Endocannabinoid Modulators: Therapeutic Promises and Challenges." *Clinical Neuroscience Research.* September 2008.

Iffland, K. et al. "An Update on Safety and Side Effects of Cannabidiol: A Review of Clinical Data and Relevant Animal Studies." *Cannabis and Cannabinoid Research.* June 2017.

Kaplan, J. et al. "Cannabidiol Attenuates Seizures and Social Deficits in a Mouse Model of Dravet Syndrome." *Proceedings of the National Academy of Sciences.* October 2017.

Kerr, A. et al. "Marijuana Use Among Patients with Epilepsy at a Tertiary Care Center." *Epilepsy & Behavior*. June 2019.

Pretzsch, C. et al. "The Effect of Cannabidiol (CBD) On Low-Frequency Activity and Functional Connectivity in the Brain of Adults with and without Autism Spectrum Disorder (ASD)." *Journal of Psychopharmacology*. June 2019.

Samanta, D. "Cannabidiol: A Review of Clinical Efficacy and Safety in Epilepsy." *Pediatric Neurology*. July 2019.

Silvestro, S. et al. "Use of Cannabidiol in the Treatment of Epilepsy: Efficacy and Security in Clinical Trials." *Molecules*. April 2019.

Weir, K. "Marijuana and the Developing Brain." *American Psychological Association*. November 2015.

Wolff, D. et al. "Use of Cannabidiol Oil in Children." *Nederlands Tijdschrift voor Geneeskunde*. May 2019.

215

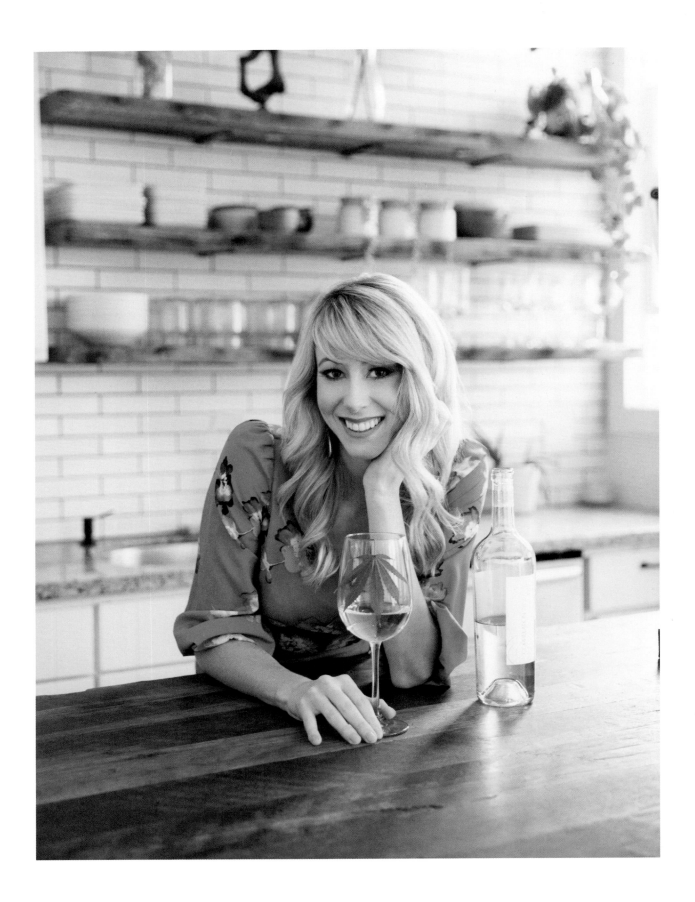

ABOUT THE AUTHOR

Jamie Evans is the founder of *The Herb Somm,* a cannabis blog and lifestyle brand that is focused on the gourmet side of the industry. She is an educator, host, and writer specializing in cannabis, CBD, food, wine, and the canna-culinary world.

As a well-known CBD and cannabis personality, Jamie has contributed to *POPSUGAR, MARY Magazine,* and *The Clever Root* magazine specializing in cannabis and CBD lifestyle features for the modern consumer. In addition, Jamie is the co-editor of GoldLeaf's acclaimed Cannabis *Cooking Journal.*

As an industry leader, Jamie was named one of *Wine Enthusiast Magazine*'s Top 40 Under 40 Tastemakers in 2018 and as a 2018 Innovator by *SevenFifty Daily,* both recognizing her efforts in the cannabis industry.

Alongside her work in the cannabis space, Jamie has more than a decade of wine industry experience. As a Certified Specialist of Wine, she continues her wine education at the San Francisco Wine School.

The Herb Somm was created in March 2017 with the goal of educating consumers and the public about cannabis, and healthy ways to incorporate herbal products into everyday life. While there is an emphasis on cannabis pairings and recipes, wellness and CBD education are naturally a focus for the brand.

ACKNOWLEDGMENTS

This book was truly a team effort! First, I want to thank my parents, Nancy and Jim Evans, who've always been my biggest cheerleaders. Your continued support means the world to me and I am happy that you've both found a place for cannabis and CBD in your self-care routines. I love you.

I want to thank my husband, Stratos Christianakis, who believed in me when I quit my full-time job to pursue my dreams in cannabis. Without your support, The Herb Somm would not exist today. I also want to thank you for helping me edit this book. Your deep wisdom about cannabis and CBD is truly remarkable. I love you.

A big thank you to my sister, Kayla, and brother-in-law, Mishka, who first came up with the name, The Herb Somm. Your creative minds continue to inspire me. Thank you to my extended families, The Barbers, The Evans, The Christianakis, and The Vom Dorps, for your support and believing in my vision. I love you.

I want to thank my editor, Thom O'Hearn, for reaching out to me with the idea of creating a CBD book. It's been an honor and a pleasure to work with you. Dreams really do come true. What an incredible project this has been! Thank you so much. I also want to thank my Project Manager, Meredith Quinn. I am so grateful for your direction and help with this book. Thank you! Also, a big shout out to my wonderful copyeditor, Jenna Patton, for helping me refine this labor of love.

Thank you to Quarto Publishing Group and Fair Winds Press for being such a wonderful publishing house to work with. This book has been a blessing, and I am eternally grateful for the opportunity to share CBD education with the world.

A big shout out and thank you to my photographer, Colleen Eversman, who shot the photos for this book. You rock, sister! I am blown away by your talent and charm.

Thank you to David Martinell and Quarto's design team who made my vision come to life. This book is so beautiful. Thank you!

A heartfelt thank you to my wonderful expert contributors including Dr. Shivani Amin, Dr. Michele Ross, Charlotte Palermino, Marcia Gagliardi, Elise McRoberts, Gillian Levy, John Korkidis, Rachel Burkons, Warren Bobrow, Monica Lo, Yannick Crespo, Chef Coreen Carroll, Chef Holden Jagger, Chef Calvin Eng, Amanda Howland, Kimberly Dillon, Claudia Mata, Dee Dussault, Cyo Nystrom, and Rachel Washtien. You are all pioneers in this industry and I am beyond grateful for the information that you were willing to share. Cheers to you all.

Last but not least, I want to thank my wonderful readers and fans who have believed in my work from the very beginning. I am so grateful for your support and for this community.

Peace, love & cannabis.

INDEX